THE SACRED BODY

MW01251205

THE SACRED BODY

A THERAPIST'S JOURNEY

MAVIS HIMES

Stoddart

Copyright © 2002 by Mavis Himes

All rights reserved. No part of this publication may be reproduced
or transmitted in any form or by any means, electronic or mechanical,
including photocopying, recording, or any information storage and retrieval system,
without permission in writing from the publisher.

Published in 2002 by
Stoddart Publishing Co. Limited
895 Don Mills Road, 400-2 Park Centre, Toronto, Canada M3C 1W3
PMB 128, 4500 Witmer Estates, Niagara Falls, New York 14305-1386

www.stoddartpub.com

To order Stoddart books please contact General Distribution Services
In Canada Tel. (416) 213-1919 Fax (416) 213-1917
Email cservice@genpub.com
In the United States Toll-free tel. 1-800-805-1083 Toll-free fax 1-800-481-6207
Email gdsinc@genpub.com

10 9 8 7 6 5 4 3 2 1

National Library of Canada Cataloguing in Publication Data
Himes, Mavis Carole, 1950–
The sacred body: a therapist's journey
ISBN 0-7737-6276-0
1. Cancer — Psychological aspects. 2. Cancer — Patients — Rehabilitation. 3.
Himes, Mavis Carole, 1950–. 4. Psychotherapists — Canada — Biography. I. Title.

RC261.H55 2002 616.99'4'0019 C2002-900577-9

**U.S. Cataloging-in-Publication Data
Available from the Library of Congress**

Cover design: Angel Guerra
Text design: Tannice Goddard

THE CANADA COUNCIL FOR THE ARTS SINCE 1957 | LE CONSEIL DES ARTS DU CANADA DEPUIS 1957

We acknowledge for their financial support of our publishing program the Canada Council, the Ontario Arts Council, and the Government of Canada through the Book Publishing Industry Development Program (BPIDP).

Printed and bound in Canada

for
all the members of Wellspring,
and in memory of
Sid and Gita

ACKNOWLEDGEMENTS

My first debt of gratitude goes to the members of Wellspring and all the men and women living with cancer who have taught me invaluable lessons in life.

Among the numerous people who have encouraged me along the way, a few names stand out. I would like to mention Austin Clarke, who taught me that one must finish what one starts, and who urged me to complete the manuscript of this book when it was still in its embryonic stage. I would also like to thank my first reader, Sam Solecki, for his astute comments, helpful suggestions, and support. Similarly, I would like to thank Lynda Morrison and Anne Hampson for their ongoing enthusiasm and support for my writing.

Conversations with several individuals have enriched my

knowledge of specific material in the text. To this end, I would like to acknowledge Dr. Manuel Buchwald, Dr. Mitchell Brown, Rabbi Elyse Goldstein, Holly Bradley, Peter Bogart, and Doris Howell.

To Don Bastian, managing editor at Stoddart, I wish to express my heartfelt appreciation for trusting his intuition and having faith in this project. To Steven Beattie, my editor, whose persistent optimism and enthusiasm encouraged me from beginning to end, my thanks for respecting my words and keeping me always on schedule. And to Gillian Watts, my gratefulness for a job well done.

Finally, I wish to express my very deepest thanks to Lawlor, my husband and soulmate, whose never-ending love and confidence in me and my work have nourished me throughout the process. And ditto for Jesse.

Author's Note: To protect their privacy and anonymity, the names of all members of Wellspring have been changed.

INTRODUCTION

For most of us, our days are spent in ritualized behaviors: complaining about the cold, frigid days of winter or July heat waves, walking the dog or feeding the cat, putting out the garbage and worrying about meal plans, balancing budgets and satisfying our employers at work or our most valued charges at home. Most of us walk or drive to work along routes that have become familiar and routine, sleep on the same side of the bed and sit at the same place at the kitchen table that we have for years, and fold our sheets and towels in particular ways, usually like our mothers or, perhaps, our lovers. We live in self-prescribed ways and are more often than not caught up in the minutiae of daily living, trapped in the growing pains of our rapidly expanding technology and preoccupation with our economic plight.

Most of us do not often stop to question these automatic patterns or to ponder the meaning of our daily lives, let alone the broad questions of the universe that intrigue philosophers, mystics, and scientists. Instead, we live our lives in segments of time, dividing our day into a pie graph of work, leisure, and sleep, while satisfying ourselves with a diet of pleasure, comfort, and rest.

Some of us are fortunate enough to carry on this way for years, even for a lifetime. But some are shocked into a major life change by personal tragedy — an accident, a sudden death, diagnosis of a life-threatening illness — an unanticipated event that disrupts our imperfect but well-ordered personal universe. And like a falling house of cards, this trauma sends shock waves not only through our own psychic being, but expanding out to others — family, friends, and colleagues — with whom we share our lives. This trauma has the potential to shatter our lives and wreak havoc on our relationships. At the same time, within it lies a seed with the potential for new growth. In the midst of psychic chaos and upheaval, one is forced to evaluate (or re-evaluate) one's life, to examine profound questions about one's connection to family, to friends, to God and the cosmos. In popular terminology, this is the famous "wake-up call."

Cancer, euphemistically called "the Big C," is one of those illnesses that cause seismic trembling in our psychic landscape. There is something so powerful about it that its very name evokes a shudder in each and every one of us. Even children who have had no contact with the disease know there is something scary and dangerous about it. And most of us can remember our first personal experience of a loved one's being diagnosed with cancer.

Is it that we still associate cancer with the inevitability of death? Or do we continue to keep it in the same box as leprosy, as something to be shunned, contained, lest it contaminate us? Is there some stigma that turns rational human beings, known for their wit, humor, psychological acumen, and intellectual prowess, into societal pariahs once they are diagnosed? Do primitive beliefs and superstition continue to dominate our thinking when we are confronted with the reality of cancer?

Cancer is clearly a signifier of mythic proportion, too big for any individual to ignore. It inscribes itself not only upon our bodies, but also in our minds. It is not uncommon to hear that once you have cancer, you can never go back to being the person you were before the diagnosis. For some, the change is minor, a small blip in their outlook. For others, dramatic changes result that involve complete personal reappraisal and a departure from former lifestyles. In other words, the diagnosis becomes a catalyst for a personal journey, a unique journey that may be shared with others, in a group or in therapy, or experienced alone.

My experience with cancer began with my family. On my paternal side, of nine brothers and sisters, five died from heart disease (including my father) and two from cancer; the remaining two siblings are still alive. On my maternal side, both my grandmother and my mother were twice diagnosed with breast cancer and, most recently, my sister was diagnosed with in situ breast cancer, a very early form of the disease. Outside my immediate family, more distant maternal great-aunts and cousins also carried this disease within their genetic code.

As a practicing psychologist for twenty-five years, I encountered several patients who were diagnosed with cancer during the course of their therapy. When I first began practicing, I specialized in the area of child and adolescent psychology. I worked in a number of different children's mental health clinics, including two years abroad in Israel. Later, I moved into psychoanalytic work with adults.

In addition to my full-time work, for ten years I was involved as a volunteer with Bereaved Families of Ontario in a variety of capacities: as chair of the Children's Program, as chair of the Professional Advisory Committee, and as a member of the board, throughout this time also facilitating groups for bereaved children. In my work I met children whose mother or father, sister or brother had died of cancer, I listened to spouses talking about a partner's death from cancer, I gave workshops on bereavement and loss, I counseled many bereaved individuals, and I studied the literature on bereavement.

In 1987 I accepted the position of acting director at Wellspring, a newly formed support center for cancer patients and their families in Toronto. And it was at Wellspring that I truly learned about the cancer experience and what it meant for individuals and their families living with cancer.

In my capacity as program director, I developed and organized a schedule of programs that continue to be offered today. These include such diverse activities as art therapy, therapeutic touch, yoga, journaling, and specialized support groups for young people, children, and patients living with metastatic disease. During that time, I also facilitated a number of newly established support groups in order to ensure that they were appropriate for the program roster.

After two years as director, I resigned in order to return to my full-time psychotherapy practice, as the job had become more administrative and less clinical. However, I continued (and still continue to the present day) to facilitate groups at Wellspring, particularly the group for people with metastatic disease and the group for young adults. In addition, I am involved in the training of volunteers who provide peer support and who co-facilitate the groups.

In spite of my previous clinical and personal experience with cancer, my background, and my professional training, I was surprised at the impact this work had on me. Nothing had prepared me for the emotional strain and pain of working with this population. In time, I began to realize that not only do cancer patients proceed through what Dr. Alastair Cunningham calls a "healing journey," but there is also a parallel process unwittingly engaged in by the therapists who help them. As a colleague of mine once said, "The struggle of being with those who are suffering is also our struggle."

As a psychologist and analyst, I became interested in the unconscious processes created by the diagnosis of cancer. I was curious about the conscious and unconscious meanings of cancer in people's lives and how unconscious fantasies about their bodies and the illness affected their psychological functioning. I was engaged in helping people to develop coping skills and to come to terms with this disease, but as a professional and as a human being, I was not myself immune to the terror of cancer. Like the members of my groups, I too had to face my medical history, my anxieties about illness, death, and dying. I too was forced to confront my beliefs about alternative medicine, radical treatments, the causes of cancer — and their implications for cure or healing. I too was challenged in my convictions about the meaning of life and the place of suffering, religion, and god in that belief system.

As I began to talk about my work with friends and colleagues, I was struck by the consistency of the questions they asked. "How do you do this work?" "Isn't it so depressing?" "How do you cope with all that suffering and loss?" These questions began to plague me, and eventually became the basis for this book. As I started to consider my own motives and interest in this type of work, I found myself thinking about my family's medical history. I quickly realized that my professional story was directly linked to my medical autobiography, and that my own inner turbulence mirrored that of the cancer patients to whom I was listening. I soon discovered that I had no magical solutions for cancer patients, or for my colleagues. Instead, as I developed my own understanding of life and challenged my own belief systems, I became able to hear stories of chaos without demanding a resolution. In this way I could cope with pain in others without feeling the need to rescue them.

Just as cancer patients are advised to do, I continued to push myself to explore in writing my journey through this work. In sharing the resulting product, I hope that other professionals will become aware of the parallels between our own journeys and those of our patients. As professionals, we do not like to expose our vulnerabilities or lose our emotional distance. Nor would it be particularly helpful to discuss our own fears and anxieties in a group or individual session. Yet we are human, and bound to become overwhelmed by the repeated stories of pain, the reminders of the cruelty of cancer and the seeming injustice of fate. And so we are pushed back, again and again, into the soul-searching that helps us remain available to listen.

At first this book was intended primarily for professionals and students working in the cancer field — doctors, nurses, social workers, psychologists, educators, clergy, and so forth — and also secondarily for those involved in the care of cancer patients and others with life-threatening diseases. But as I continued to write and share my writing with others, I realized that it should be shared also with the general public, as we are all touched by cancer, whether directly or indirectly. Perhaps, in a more grandiose way, I hope that this book will also demystify fears about the disease known as the Big C, and be of interest to both those who are living with cancer and those who are not. I hope that it will inspire readers to examine their own beliefs about life and death.

It was not my purpose to write a psychological how-to book of coping techniques and tools, or a spiritual book of guidelines and magical formulae for cure or health. Instead, this book is a memoir that traces the personal journey of one therapist and, if it challenges others to similarly look inward, then I will be satisfied that I have accomplished my aim.

1

I come from a family that is blended in a medical marriage of heart disease and cancer. Of my father's eight brothers and sisters, five died from heart attacks (including my father) and two from cancer, and the two remaining siblings battle high cholesterol and clogged arteries. My mother says their pores have been saturated by a diet of chicken fat and pickled tongue, beef brisket and schmaltz herring, cheese kreplach and potato latkes, that they brought with them from Minsk and Radauti. Their Russian-Rumanian bellies fasted on the meager rations of the war years and feasted in the years of plenty.

"They're big eaters," my slim mother would say. "Big eaters and rich foods. Look at Ida's waistline — bulging at the seams."

I learned early on that the Himes physical genotype was not to be emulated.

Both my paternal grandparents died before I was born. My grandfather was born in Radauti, Rumania, in 1880. In 1910 or thereabouts, he immigrated to Canada, where he subsequently married my grandmother, Annie Chernofsky, a girl of eighteen. My grandmother was born in Minsk, Russia, and had immigrated to Canada with her parents sometime between 1904 and 1908, during one of the periods of Russian pogroms.

I have a photocopied photograph of my grandfather when he was in his early sixties. Morris Heimovitch had blond hair and blue eyes. In the picture, his hair looks white and his upper lip is lined with a thin moustache. In the photograph of my grandmother, Annie Chernofsky Heimovitch, she is holding a baby in her arms, while two other children cling to either side of her full-length skirt. I think the baby is my father, but he is no longer alive to confirm this.

My father was exceedingly secretive about his childhood and shied away from any conversations I initiated on the topic. As a result, the information for the biographical scrapbook of my family has been cut and pasted from conversations with my Aunt Ida and my cousin Andrea, from the family tree begun by my cousin Melvin, and from my own musings.

My father's original name was Louis Frank Heimovitch. A 1915 census of Montreal shows that he grew up at 62 Grubert Lane, in a crowded Jewish neighborhood. Nine brothers and sisters were tucked into a two-bedroom flat with a back-alley entrance atop a dozen or more metal stairs. Morris, my grandfather, had no technical skills or trade. Like many other immigrants, he peddled wares on "the Main" immortalized by Mordecai Richler. As Morris wheeled his pushcart up and down Saint-Laurent Boulevard, my grandmother stayed home, bent over a pot of potatoes and onions, stirring in love and what little nutrition was available to feed the hungry mouths of Phil and Harry and Louis and Ida and Percy and Hymie and Betty and Leonard and Meyer. As each of the boys reached secondary-school age, he ended his education in order to supplement the family means. The girls stayed home to help their mother.

My father was an outgoing man. His extroversion, so unlike my mother's cool reserve, shone through his lustrous eyes and broad smile. Raised in an orthodox Jewish home by an ignorant yet religious autocrat, my father and his eight siblings learned from an early age the meanings of both work and faith. And my grandfather expected that my father, as one of the older boys, would be a role model for the others.

All the boys were forced to work. Work was what you had to do to stay alive, to survive, to put potatoes and eggs on the table. But faith was the true master, the raison d'être of life. Without faith, there would be no meaning, and without meaning, there would be no purpose to getting up and making ready for the day, to walking five kilometers to synagogue at dawn in order to thank God for another day, another blessing.

In my father's family, there could be no such luxury as rebellion, as adolescent insurrection. In moments of rage at minor infractions of devotion, my grandfather would quietly but forcefully say, "See this strap? Kiss it. Kiss the strap." He was ruled by devotion and obedience, and demanded the same from his children. Judaism as interpreted through my grandfather's eyes was a religion of fear, not of compassion.

My paternal grandmother, who spent most of her time in pregnancy and childbirth, also dreaded the steely blue eyes of my austere grandfather. Fifteen years his junior, timid Annie Chernofsky was forced into an arranged marriage when she was eighteen. Unlike my grandfather, who came from a small town, my grandmother was a big-city girl, the daughter of a self-taught man. Much like the reign of terror my grandfather wielded over the boys, my grandparents' marriage was characterized by dominance and submission.

Six nights a week, Annie boiled vegetables: beets for borscht, potatoes for cholent, carrots and celery and turnips for soup, cabbage for stuffed *holishkes*. And once a week, she prepared a special Shabbat meal for her husband and children. On the table were a white embroidered tablecloth inherited from her mother, a pair of silver candlesticks, and a silver bread plate with a hand-embroidered cover for the challah.

The children emerged from their regular activities, scrubbed clean and dressed in their Shabbat clothes. As my grandmother, surrounded by her brood, lit the Shabbat candles, she beamed with pride. What was the hardship of the week, the penny-pinching, the scraping, the words of abuse, compared to the joy and *naches* of having produced nine such healthy children? No matter that all her working hours were devoted to shopping and cooking and cleaning, that her legs were puffed up with edema and poor circulation, that her body had swelled and shrunk with regular childbearing for almost nine consecutive years, or that her husband could at times be an animal. She would close her eyes, warming herself with the flame of family and home, and murmur the words of blessing over the candles — *Baruch atah adonai elohenu melech ha'olam* . . . For those few short hours, Annie Heimovitch felt at peace.

As the Heimovitch boys grew up, the spirit of survival with which they had been indoctrinated was redirected into their work. My father, demonstrating social talents from an early age, was well liked by many people, who subsequently helped him with work. He began with a number of odd jobs: short-order cook, factory shipper, hot-dog vendor. In 1945, he and a friend from Baron Byng High School founded what would become a successful women's clothing company. By his late twenties, my father was well established in the garment industry.

Sometime during this period, the Heimovitch brothers "shortened" their name to Himes — for business purposes, my father told me. Perhaps they wanted to become more assimilated into the Montreal of the forties. Perhaps they wanted to be separate — marked apart from the Jews with long sideburns, black fedoras, and long black topcoats, those strange-looking men with anemic complexions who scurried to and fro in the passageways of the market on Friday afternoons before sunset. Perhaps they wanted to be able to mix anonymously with the crowds on Sherbrooke and Dorchester streets and up and down the aisles of Ogilvy's, with its plaid boxes and its heraldic coat of arms in the foyer. Perhaps they wished to go unnoticed, unrecognized for who they were — the Heimovitch boys from the Main.

In 1945, the same year that my father founded his company, he married my mother, Miriam Rabinovitch, the only child of

Hymie and Bertha Rabinovitch. That same year also, my father became an orphan when his mother died in her early fifties of unknown causes; his father had died in 1942. It is said that when Annie Chernofsky Heimovitch closed her eyes that Friday night, she was finally at peace.

In spite of his newly acquired emancipation, my father's strong ethnic identity still branded him an Old World icon. Born in a tenement in Montreal's Jewish ghetto, he had left this familiar territory a few years after he married, moving with his contemporaries to the uptown suburbs. Yet every morning he would return to work in the neighborhood of his past, mixing with his landsmen of Rumanian and Russian descent. And every evening he would return to the manicured lawns of suburban Hampstead.

In my mother, Louis Himes had found a trophy of beauty, elegance, and charm. Shamefully hiding his impoverished background from the woman he had married, he embraced my mother's ambitions of wealth. Together they formed a perfect duo, combining my mother's sense of aesthetics and my father's financial success. Slowly they established a residence full of finery, good taste, and haute culture.

The Museum, which is what my sister, Linda, and I christened the house, was a continuous work in progress. There was always more to be done — more walls to be painted, more furniture to be ordered from New York, more floors to be stained, more paintings and sculpture to collect. One week, when my father was out of town on a business trip, my mother had the center post of the basement replaced by a ceiling beam. I remember her immediately demanding approval. "I'm not sure why your father never wanted to remove that ugly thing. It ruined the space. I'm sure he thought the room would collapse if we removed it. So now, don't you agree it looks better?" One couldn't deny the room's increased openness, yet Linda and I both felt a certain tenderness and loyalty toward my father's insistence on the status quo.

From my limited perspective as a child, I always saw my mother as the leader and my father as follower. And yet, in spite of their differences, they enjoyed a happy marriage. My father was proud of my mother's talents as a "lady of the house," admonishing my sister and I to take note of them. And my mother respected and appreciated my father's devotion to his family, a devotion that he had transferred from an invisible god to a beautiful queen.

• • •

"You kids are all spoiled," my father would say regularly. "When we were your age, we made up our own games — no need for all these fancy toys." Linda and I would roll our eyes. We indulged like other children in a make-believe world full of dolls and stuffed animals, brought home successful report cards, and earned praise and the reward of our parents' affection.

But when I was an adolescent, the childhood romance with my father ended. He and I butted heads daily. Philosophy, education, politics — any topic could incite heated words. A self-taught man, my father mistrusted the books of higher learning, yet insisted that his daughters be educated. There was no question about education; the questions were *where* and *what.*

"You may have a university degree, fancy-shmancy books, but what do you know about making a living? You can't eat your books!" he would shout.

In retaliation, I fought back with my own choice words. "Karl Marx says . . . Spinoza says . . ."

"And who paid for those words? Who gave you the opportunity to go to university and smoke marijuana with all those longhairs? Don't think I don't know what goes on there!"

Stalemate. Exit to my bedroom.

I studied psychology in university. There I met a man who swept me off my feet with his lofty words and his full beard, low-slung jeans, and army coat. Serge was seductive. In the kitchen, my mother glared at him out of the corner of her eye.

Serge worked in the psychology lab seven nights a week doing research. McGill University was well-known for its focus on academic psychology, particularly in the subjects of motivation, perception, and physiology. Donald Hebb, whose classic text we would regurgitate in Psychology 101, warned his five hundred freshmen students in September, "If you think psychology is going to help you learn to analyze your friends, then you might as well leave now." We all looked around at each other and took out our pens, ready to begin taking notes. "Today we will ask the questions, Why psychology? What psychology? Why comparative ethology? . . ."

I didn't bother to save my notes from those early courses, or my essays on motivation trends in primates, classical conditioning versus operant learning, thought and language in preschoolers, and paradigms of experimental design. I didn't take much interest in animal behavior, statistics, or abnormal behavior. Instead I followed the young man with the low-slung jeans and the Leonidas boots.

Serge worked in the lab on the ninth floor stimulating the amygdalas of cats; that part of the brain is considered to be the center of aggression. Serge was two years ahead of me. When he left to carry on graduate work at the University of Western Ontario, I picked up where he left off, studying the behavioral correlates of aggression in rats. Seven days a week, I took a bus to the lab in the Medical Sciences Building, observed the attack strategies of food-deprived black-hooded rats, and weighed the remains of the mice they had killed. When the study was over, I had to euthanize all the animals I had used. Contaminated for future studies, their brief lives had been dedicated to the cause of science. Today I wince at the thought of all those animals sacrificed for the sake of scientific discovery.

When Serge and I ended our relationship during my third year, I ended my studies in animal research. My fourth-year honors thesis was on laughter and humor in children. There I discovered another side of psychological research: the human subject. I subsequently went on to do graduate work in psychology and moved into the clinical arena of working with people.

As a student intern, I worked with children whose families were unable to provide them with the necessary warmth, affection, and background to develop into mature and healthy individuals. I practiced as a child psychotherapist, talking and listening to boys and girls as we played with a dollhouse, puppets, dinosaurs, and trains. I tried to create an environment in which it was safe to act out and discuss life's imperfections.

Unfortunately, my father never understood the premise of psychology: providing others with a forum to help them work out their problems. Or perhaps he simply chose to ignore its usefulness as a profession. "A helping profession? Who gets help?" he would ask. I sensed an irrational quality to my father's frustration with my chosen profession. He was certainly not the kind of man to open his heart to strangers. He was of a generation in which problems stayed locked within the privacy of the family. Only *meshugenahs*, the crazy ones, went to a psychiatrist.

When I graduated, however, my father overcame his reservations and was quick to introduce me with pride: "Meet my daughter, the doctor." In his fantasy, I suppose I was a medical practitioner, not someone who played with people's minds.

Many years later, I learned some family history from my Aunt Ida, my father's sister with the bulging waistline and broad hips, who went to McGill in her sixties to complete an undergraduate degree in political science. She told me that when she was young, her parents had been visited by social workers who attempted to offer the family financial assistance. The Heimovitch brothers refused help. "Charity? We are not a charity case." The door of 62 Grubert Lane was slammed on the lady in the stiff white shirt and thick-soled shoes.

• • •

My father's first heart attack occurred when I was ten years old. My parents had returned from an evening out at their golf and country club. It was ten o'clock on a Wednesday night, and my sister and I were sleeping while my grandmother was downstairs watching television. My mother called out that my dad wasn't feeling well, that he had indigestion or something. Her voice was taut, verging on a shriek. When my sister and I ran out of our bedroom, she told us to go back to bed and be quiet.

I remember lying in bed and hearing my father trudge up and down the stairs from midnight on, while my mother tried to persuade him to lie down or call the doctor. I fell asleep with the sound of my father's footsteps in my dreams. In the morning, Dr. Rodin, our handsome family physician with the wavy auburn hair and a number tattooed on his forearm, rang the doorbell. My mother, wrapped in my father's terry-cloth robe, answered the door. Her face blotchy and white, she ushered the doctor into their bedroom, where my father's body lay in a heap under the sheets, his chest heaving spasmodically. Dr. Rodin entered and shut the door behind him.

Within ten minutes of the doctor's arrival, an ambulance screamed into our driveway. My father was wheeled out of the house on a gurney. I tried to restrain myself from tears. As if forewarned, a crowd of neighbors instantly lined the sidewalk, and, no longer able to contain my sobs, I burst out screaming, "Go home, go home! Get away from here!" Linda took my hand and gave it a squeeze. "It's going to be okay. They're just taking him to the hospital." I didn't believe her.

My father survived that first heart attack, as well as the next two. I once read in a newspaper that if you survive seven heart attacks, you're home free. I wonder if "home free" takes on a different meaning if you're religious — such as leaving the world of earthly possessions to be reunited with God in another home.

Twenty-two years after his first coronary, my father's heart gave out and he was finally home free. He had been dancing with my mother on New Year's Eve while on holiday in Miami Beach. Prior to his trip, his cardiologist had given him the medical stamp of approval. "Go and enjoy yourself. Just remember to keep up the daily exercise — and no cheesecake." Maybe his doctor thought he was home free, too.

My mother says, "Your dad was always in a hurry. See, even when it comes to living his life, he's in a rush for the finish line."

The night my dad died, I was adrift — floating on a sea of champagne bubbles and caviar, awash in love, enamored of the new man in my life. Streamers and balloons filled the dimly lit restaurant. For me, this New Year's Eve was a toast as much to a newly created union of love as it was to the new year.

The night my dad died, I was wearing a sexy black dress with sequins and a low-cut back. Lawlor held my hand under the table. Furtively, like adolescents, we exchanged amorous glances, pretending we were carrying on a secret tryst, meeting in a dark trattoria to preserve our anonymity. Around us, people were oblivious to our game. We drank, we danced, we cajoled, we ate, we laughed. We made our private declaration of love in a public place.

"I love you *this* much," said Lawlor, indicating with his hands the broad sweep of the room.

"And I love you forever and ever," I retorted, giddy from the sparkling fizz.

"But show me how much," he demanded. I gestured the moon and the stars and the earth and the four directions of the winds. And then I stood up, leaned forward on unsteady feet, and planted a big red kiss on his cheek. We left early, singing and glowing. Embroidered snowflakes landed on our cheeks, melting on contact. We toasted in silence our love and good fortune.

I hated it that Lawlor was leaving for the airport. I had refused his repeated invitations to join him on a trip to Mexico to see his daughter and newly born granddaughter. Suddenly, I regretted my decision; I didn't want him to leave. I said goodbye with tears in my eyes as he dropped me off at my apartment. Then I collapsed on the bed, disconnected the phone, and fell asleep.

The night my dad died, he was at the Hotel Fontainebleau in Miami Beach. He was wearing his navy blue suit, the one that made him look so handsome, that set off his white hair, the one I loved so much. He was dancing with my mother, surrounded by friends from Montreal.

The night my dad died, he was walking off the dance floor, accompanying my mother back to their table, when he collapsed. He collapsed and my mother shrieked and Evelyn Stein spilt red wine on the white linen tablecloth and Eddy Wagman tripped as he ran over to my father. Within seconds, I am told, a crowd had circled him, and a doctor in the group pushed people away to make room and the ambulance arrived and my mother sat in the front of it praying under her breath and rifling her purse and the ambulance men asked her if she wanted a tissue. When they arrived at the hospital, she told me later, my mother already knew that my dad was dead.

The night my dad died, TV broadcasters were reviewing the major events of the year. Princess Grace had been killed in an automobile crash. Yassir Arafat had signed a declaration accepting Israel's right to exist. The New York Islanders had beaten

Vancouver for the Stanley Cup. Bertha Wilson had become the first woman to be appointed a justice of the Supreme Court of Canada.

I flew to Montreal for the funeral. When I got to the house on Queen Mary Road, my mother had not yet arrived back from Florida. I ran up the stairs to get some tissues from the washroom. I shrieked. A puddle of red nail polish lay on the green bath mat sitting so innocently on the black tiles in the middle of the room. My mother returned a few hours later.

The Torah states ". . . dust you are and to dust shall you return" (Gen. 3:19). As the deceased cannot obey the commandment to return to dust, the family arranges it for him or her. The traditional flimsy coffin is designed to speed decomposition of the body — its return to the earth. Sometimes Jews were buried only in a cloth shroud in direct contact with the soil.

A leading authority, Rabbi Leo Trepp, writes in his book on Jewish observances,

> Many peoples of antiquity surrounded a funeral with great ceremony. In Egypt the annual funeral of Osiris lasted for seven days, and Jews have a similar period of deep mourning. Grief was powerfully expressed and even induced by professional "lamenters," women who raised their voices in agonizing shrieks, tore their hair and garments, and sometimes incised their bodies. Incisions are forbidden by Torah. Public lamentation was an accepted part of ancient funeral rites.

I no longer remember the funeral ceremony, the words of praise, the prayers uttered by the rabbi. I remember only a sea of bobbing heads and my own cold hands and feet. Following the service, we piled out into the glaring sunshine of an icy January day. I dropped my sunglasses, accidentally crushing them under my boots. The cars were black and the upholstery was black and my mother's scarf was black. I saw a black crow land on a telephone wire as we approached the cemetery in the eastern section of Montreal.

When all were assembled, there were more prayers and more tears and more tissues. I was the third to drop earth on the coffin, after my mother and sister. Then the rest of the mourners helped to fill the grave, shaping the mound. There was no deception — the end had come.

For the next seven days, during the traditional ritual of shivah, my hand was repeatedly shaken, my body hugged over and over again. I looked quizzically at the people who so intimately pronounced my name. "So, *you're* Mavis. I've heard so much about you from your father." People swarmed the house and every night I plummeted into a deep chasm of sleep.

When the seven days were over, I left Montreal. I left the photographs, the drawers of sweaters, the shoes neatly lined up in rows, the ordered collection of ties hanging behind the bedroom door. I left my father's house with its tapestry of a northern Quebec village, the shelves of Inuit sculpture, the pottery vases, the wall-sized painting by Jack Shadbolt, a lifetime's accumulation of souvenirs and mementos. I left my childhood home in which I no longer felt like a child.

I returned to Toronto by rail. In spite of Lawlor's ministrations of love and support, I felt submerged in a black space, paralyzed and immobile. I did not cry for several months; my tear ducts were frozen. In my dreams, I cried and cried, waking with puffy eyelids, but during the day, I moved to and fro between house and office in a trance. I stopped eating. I stopped sleeping. I went to see a psychiatrist. The blackness slowly turned into a thick gray fog that settled inside me for months before it gradually lifted.

Memories flooded my thoughts: the first time he took me skiing, when he wore a black-and-white toque that I teased him about; my tenth birthday, when he took three friends and me on a sleigh ride up Mount Royal; the shuffling of his slippers on the kitchen floor; the creases beside his laughing eyes; the time he congratulated me on my first university degree; dancing my first cha-cha with him at my cousin Murray's bar mitzvah . . .

I began to see my father every time I saw the back of a white-haired man of his height. I pulled out photo albums to hold on to the legacy of shared memories we had created.

A memory. Every *erev* Rosh Hashanah, the eve of the Jewish New Year, my father and I would walk to synagogue together. Neither my mother nor my sister went to synagogue; only my father and I would quietly rise from the table, its white tablecloth stained with red wine and sprinkled with crumbs of honey cake, scramble out the front door, and wind our way through the neighborhood streets hand in hand. The ring on his pinky squeezed my fingers painfully, but I never complained. His hand would be warm and he would smell of spicy limes. My father would be wearing his navy suit and shiny Italian shoes. He would carry his blue velvet *tallit* bag in his free hand and I would feel proud to be seen with him. I would be wearing a new outfit bought specially for the holidays. My father never wore his yarmulke as we walked; he always waited until we had gone through the oak doors of the synagogue before placing it on his head.

Once inside, we would separate. He would go off with his friends from the congregation and sit in a section reserved for the men only. I would inevitably meet my girlfriends and we would sit in the women's section on the unnumbered seats in the balcony, or at the very back of the chapel, where wooden bridge-chairs had been added for the High Holiday services. My father and I would reunite after the service, wishing each other and everyone else in the crowded lobby a happy new year. As the crowds of people dispersed, my father and I would walk back home, tired and unhurried.

My last memory. My father was in Toronto for a business trip and we agreed to get together later in the day. He met me at my workplace, a children's mental health clinic where I saw emotionally troubled preschoolers. I introduced my father to the staff who were still around at the end of the day and gave him a tour of the clinic. Then we drove to my apartment so that he could see my new place. I wondered what he would think of the purple bathroom. "Novel," he said, peering into the tiny room.

Because there was not much time before his flight, we decided to eat near the airport. My father sat facing me. We had never before been out together without my mother. Words did not come easily at first. I had never been particularly open or communicative with my father, especially since moving to Toronto after my undergraduate years. We talked about work, his and mine. We talked about my sister, my mother. We talked about my years overseas. And then it shifted slightly. There was a loosening, and I began to talk about my dreams, my hopes, my fears.

"I am tired of being single again. I really do hope I meet someone in the near future."

"You know, I worry about you sometimes. Being single, I mean. I guess I'm still an old traditionalist. A father just wants to see his daughter married so that he can know she is being taken care of."

"I always knew that about you, Dad. All that talk of being liberal, youthful — you're just an old chauvinist." We both laughed. The evening was too short. We had to rush to make his flight.

A week later my mother told me what a wonderful time my father had with me. "He says that he must make a point of doing that more often, having a visit with you in Toronto," she said. "He said he really got to learn about his daughter."

I said, "It was mutual. I had a great time, too. Maybe now I will be able to ask him all those questions about his family that he has always kept hidden."

My father never made it back to Toronto. He died three months later. My father never got to meet Lawlor, the man I would later marry, whom I met two weeks after our evening together. My father never got to know that I quit smoking a month later. My father never got to know who his daughter had become.

A year after my dad's death, I returned for a visit to the house I had outgrown. I crept into my parents' bedroom and peeked into my father's chest of drawers, where my mother kept some of his clothes that she could not bear to give away. One piece at a time, I took out each item of clothing. The green alpaca sweater with the Lacoste logo, which he wore to play golf. The gray cashmere V-neck sweater he wore to football games. The powder-blue shirt he wore to my graduation. The black sweater with the tufts of white wool, which he wore skiing before his first heart attack. I laid each piece gently on the bed, and then, with equal care, I put them back in their rightful spots in the drawer.

2

The room is warm today. There has been an unexpected shift in the temperature — fall is so unpredictable. I look around the room for the thermostat and notice that the side-table leg is wobbly and some magazines are about to slide off. I adjust the leg.

The women amble in, their faces shiny with perspiration. There is a buzz of activity as people get coffee and chat. I think that Sandra looks tired, and then I remember that she did not attend the group last week because of a hospital appointment. She called in crying, saying that she had received bad news and couldn't bring herself to confront the group. The faces of these women are drawn, these women who meet weekly in this spacious room at 81 Wellesley Street. They do not smile easily.

We assemble in a circle and I wait until people have settled in their chairs. Tara places her walker to one side and slides awkwardly onto the sofa. Paula is limping more than before. Maria is communicating with her interpreter, who is young and clean-cut. Maria is pointing to me. I smile hello to the young woman, whose full lips draw back in a smile. "Hello, my name is Mavis," I say to her, and then turn to the others.

"I guess we'll begin now." The women close their eyes before I say another word. The opening visualization exercise has become a welcome ritual. "Okay, then. Just begin to take some deep breaths." The words flow easily as I too relax my eyes, palms resting upward on my lap, feet planted firmly on the burgundy rug. I hear breathing — some irregular, some steady. Someone begins to cough. The door opens, and I motion for Elaine to sit down in the chair beside me.

I am never ready for this group: eight women fighting metastatic cancer.

Metastatic. An ugly word that trips up pronunciation. A paradoxical term. *Static.* There is nothing static about cancer that spreads by erupting mysteriously in new places. *Metastatic.* A word that conjures up an image of knobby joints, like the *metatarsal* bones of one's feet. But then again, why should an appealing word be used to signify such an appalling disease? What if it were a long, flowing word with sibilants and rhyming sounds? *Messasuena,* for example, would suggest something mysterious and exotic. No, perhaps the harshness of *metastatic* apt after all.

The relaxation exercise comes to an end. I ask everyone how the week has been. Sandra is sitting to my right. Today her hair is tied back at her neck with a red scarf. Her hands are weaving a pattern on her lap. "I wasn't here last week," she begins. "I had an appointment with my oncologist about my bone scan the day before. They found two new hot spots, one on my sternum and one on my pelvis. I had been complaining about a sore hip for a few weeks . . . Now I no longer qualify for a bone marrow transplant." She stops speaking.

The women listen in silence, all eyes turned on Sandra, who continues in a monotone. "I was so upset. They said it could be one of three things. First, it may be a reaction to the chemo. Second . . ." She pauses, and I watch her mouth form the words as she speaks again. ". . . the cancer may have spread." She pulls at a loose thread on her skirt. "Third, the spots were undetected in the initial scan. And if that isn't bad enough, I just learned that my long-term disability may not come through."

When Sandra elaborates on the details of her insurance claim, the other women respond immediately. "Have you called your personnel department?" "Have you called Janos at the union office? I'm a teacher too. Speak to the board office."

Sandra nods. "I have tried all that. I've been on the phone all morning and I'm all talked out right now." She keeps on nodding. In the first session, a few weeks earlier, Sandra had marveled at her condition. "I am completely asymptomatic," she said after taking me aside. "I feel too healthy. Maybe I shouldn't be in this group."

Elaine, who is sitting on my left, has been absent since the first session. I turn and ask how she has been. "I'm awful," she says, speaking as if her mouth were full of marbles. "But I am so glad to be here. I've been dreaming of your faces the past few weeks, looking forward to seeing all of you once again. I'm on my third week of chemo. I'm on taxol and it's killing me — it's just killing me." She pauses, takes a deep breath, and continues, "I don't think I can take it anymore. I've decided to go off the chemo. What kind of life is this anyway? For what? Two more months of life? Maybe six? I think I want a better quality of life."

Movement of chairs, sounds of coughing. I lose my focus. I look at Elaine and see an attractive woman a few years older than I am. Her complexion is smooth, her makeup immaculate. There is no visible sign of disease. Her hairless scalp is hidden under a felt hat with pink flowers. I think of my garden, still in bloom in late September.

Finally the silence is broken by Anika, whose eyes are puffy behind her thick-lensed glasses. "You must consult a doctor. Maybe you should see the hospital social worker. Before you make such a definite decision, you must have someone listen to your concerns."

Elaine is rolling her tongue around in her mouth and Tara offers her a lozenge. "Thanks. Maybe that's a good idea. I don't know what to do at this point. Everything aches. What's the point?"

An exchange develops, gains momentum, and then fades as Paula shares Elaine's decision-making quandary. With the intuition of a woman who has been to the edge, peered into the abyss, and returned, she says, "I am also deciding — whether to have a bone marrow transplant or to arrange palliative care. I no longer wish to buy a few months of time if it means I will be too sick to enjoy my garden. You know, the cosmos were very late to bloom this year; they have just burst forth. And the hydrangeas remind me of my childhood days. In the fall, we always went with my dad to a nursery off a country road and bought potted mums, purple cabbages, and Indian corn. I love October. . . . I have a week to decide."

• • •

Cancer. A word that conjures up images of people propped up in hospital beds, people with bald heads or stiff-looking wigs, people to be pitied for their impending deaths. *Cancer* is not a neutral word. It does not roll easily off the tongue. It sends shivers through everyone, young and old. *Cancer* is a word to which the term "anxiety" well applies — anxiety as defined by Freud, about an imminent danger from which it is impossible to escape. Cancer is clearly one such danger. The body is invaded from within, betrayed, threatened by foreign cells dividing and multiplying beyond one's control. The body, once reliable and predictable in its functioning, becomes a vault within which the malignant cells are trapped. And the skin, once a protective shield, threatens to be breached from within.

Cancer is not a fantasized illness. Its materiality is evident in the results of blood tests, ultrasounds, MRIs, body scans. It is visible in the cells with altered genes that "forget" to stop growing, eventually developing into a mass or tumor that impedes the development of healthy cells. The fears and anxieties of cancer clearly have a basis in reality. Yet dread feeds also on the fantasies of the psyche, multiplying rapidly like the rogue microscopic cells. It is often in the dark hours of the night that anxiety erupts, tightening around the stomach or head like a vise. What if I lose my mental faculties? What if I end up suffering interminably? What if I am a burden to my family?

What about the children? Will my husband remember Susie's favorite cake and what she wants for her birthday? Where will the cells attack next time?

I have read that the oldest paleopathological evidence of cancer is limited to lesions that affected bones found as fossils. Tumors have been discovered in Egyptian mummies from as far back as the third century BCE. However, it was the ancient Greeks who first familiarized themselves with this group of diseases and created a new medical category. It was Hippocrates who labeled it *karcinos* (crab).

The most common cancers were first diagnosed in women. Breast cancer is the archetypal form; its massy profile, spreading filaments, and swollen veins suggested to the Greeks the legs and feelers of a crab. This image was strengthened by other characteristics. According to one medical source, "The exterior surface was thought comparable to the texture of a crab's shell, the condition was persistent, literally refusing to let go, while the pain was like sharp claws seizing hold in the depths of the body."

Hippocratic medicine attributed tumors, which included all sorts of swellings, to abnormal accumulation of the humors. Cancer was believed to be caused by black bile, the melancholic humor. If the cancer ulcerated, the black bile was thought to be undiluted; if not, it meant the bile had been diluted. Occult (deep) growths, which were considered to be inevitably fatal, were left untreated; it was thought that the patient would live longer if the disease went untouched.

Were women more prone to melancholic humors? Was that the reason for the prevalence of breast cancer in those early days of civilization? Does today's higher incidence of depression in women compared to men contain a thread from the social fabric of the past? Or did a mutant particle infiltrate the female genetic code?

The earliest treatment of cancer was limited to such procedures as cauterization, drainage, and excision; only much later were some internal cancers treated surgically. Barber-surgeons incised and excised boils and warts as well, in the belief that they were curing cancer. It was thought at one time that cancers, at least when ulcerated, were contagious, like leprosy. Perhaps it is not surprising that many people today still cling unconsciously to this primitive belief, shunning those who are diagnosed with the disease.

The invention of microscopy revolutionized cancer research. Today cancer is treated as a modern phenomenon, one of the leading challenges facing medicine. Each year in Canada, approximately 130,000 men and women will be diagnosed with some form of cancer. They will be treated with chemotherapy, radiation therapy, surgery, or some combination of these. Depending on the type of cancer, new innovations in cancer care may be tried, such as hormone therapy for breast cancer or a stem cell transplant for multiple myeloma or lymphoma. Every day in the newspapers there are reports of new clinical trials and experimental treatments being discussed at medical forums and conferences; new and radical forms of surgery are written about in the medical journals. Some oncologists even claim that within their lifetimes chemotherapy will become extinct, replaced by newer forms of intervention.

In addition to the conventional medical treatments, within the past twenty years there has been an even more radical shift — in the field of psychoneuroimmunology, more commonly known as mind-body medicine. The work of such pioneers as Dossey, Siegel, and Simonton has been popularized by media coverage of alternative, or complementary, medicine. Today a cancer patient is faced with a multitude of choices for a treatment plan. Like a select menu of delicacies, the choices include therapeutic touch, yoga, qi gong, meditation, shark cartilage, 7-14X, chelation, omega-3, live cell therapy, astragalus, macrobiotics, and reiki, among others. In both traditional hospitals and privately funded clinics, programs such as visualization, relaxation, and art therapy are being offered. As a result, many cancer patients opt for a completely individualized program, believing that their chances for both quantity and quality of life may be improved by the addition of these adjunct therapies.

• • •

In 1901, Mary Emma Ellis sold her stately residence near the intersection of Church and Wellesley streets in Toronto to a group of businessmen for one hundred dollars. This was to be the first of a series of transactions that ultimately led to the sale of this white brick house, along with its charming coach house, to Wellspring, a center for cancer patients and their families.

Edmond George and Louis Lawrence (Bud), the Odette brothers, moved the offices of their company, Eastern Construction, into the wood-paneled rooms of Ms. Ellis's former home when they purchased the property in 1972. As Eastern Construction's profits multiplied, they outgrew the space and moved to another location. Meanwhile, Edmond, Bud, and one of their employees formed a partnership, JEB, that used the stately mansion to generate rental revenue. From 1978 to 1997, the house witnessed a number of tenants: an engineering firm, the Government of Ontario, a law office. Meanwhile, the coach house at the back was employed as the setting for various film productions.

In 1991, a petite woman in a broad-brimmed hat, whose parents were neighbors of Bud Odette, approached young Mark Odette, the property manager, about leasing the coach house for a project she had in mind, called Wellspring. (By that time, an eccentric group of criminal lawyers was occupying the offices of the main building.) The JEB partnership approved the proposal and, with a guaranteed rent, Wellspring had negotiated its first lease and moved into its first home.

I first crossed the threshold of the coach house while it was undergoing renovation. Nails and screws were scattered like the spilled contents of bins in a child's toy chest. The wind whistled through the plastic windows of the low-ceilinged living room as a group of oncologists, social workers, clinical nurse specialists, and psychologists attempted to convene amid the plaster dust and paint cans.

"The fabric was donated by the Four Seasons Hotel," I heard a woman murmur to her neighbor. "Our painter, Carl, was doing work over at Izzy Sharp's hotel, and when he heard they were going to get rid of the drapes, Carl asked if he could take them. So here we are with fifteen pairs of drapes, which will work to reupholster six sofas. And I got the chesterfields and love seats from Waddington's spring auction."

"Well, aren't you clever! That's a brilliant idea. What about checking some of the other hotels?" the woman beside her asked.

"No, I've got my eye on some furniture at Goodwill. They've promised me some good deals," the soft voice replied.

Ten minutes later, the group reassembled in a makeshift boardroom on the second floor. Fundraising, user fees, flow of patient information, grand opening event, furnishings, terms of reference — all were discussed in detail. Various models of clinical programs also came under the scrutiny of the professionals gathered in the drafty room.

I learned after the meeting that the fair-skinned woman with the black chapeau and tweed suit, whose quiet conversation about the decor I had overheard, was Anne Armstrong Gibson. She was the visionary behind those piles of planks, the sawdust, and the fifteen sets of drapes on the main floor. Anne Pollitt Armstrong Gibson — founder of Wellspring, non-Hodgkin's lymphoma patient, founder of the Genesis Research Foundation, estate lawyer, classical thinker, and animal lover. Anne Pollitt Armstrong Gibson — role model of a warrior woman to a generation of professionals, volunteers, and cancer patients who were to cross the threshold of 81 Wellesley Street East. She was a tightly wound, tenacious, and obstinate visionary who, in the spring of 1992, led her battalion of dedicated trustees and professional advisors in a victory march when Wellspring opened its freshly painted entrance to the first group of cancer patients and their families.

I had been leading groups for bereaved children through Bereaved Families of Ontario since my father's death in 1982. One day, I received a call from a colleague at Bereaved Families.

"How would you like to be on the professional advisory committee of a new cancer center that is being formed, called Wellspring? They are looking for someone who can address issues related to children and adolescents."

The first meeting I attended was held in the boardroom of Princess Margaret Hospital a few months before that site meeting. I arrived a few minutes late, as the introductions were being made, and slipped into a chair beside a handsome man with wavy salt-and-pepper hair. The men and women assembled around the table announced their credentials with confidence: senior oncologists, medical researchers, chairmen of medical teams, university department heads, psychosocial oncology specialists, a dean of nursing. The names and positions intimidated me, and when it came to my turn, I stumbled through my words. This distinguished group was to act as advisors to a new and exciting project that would revolutionize cancer care in Toronto. After the introductions, we argued, discussed, hashed, and rehashed the organizational chart, the role of the advisory committee, a proposal for basic services, representation, and the terms of reference. Everyone participated with enthusiasm and I found myself swept up in the boundless energy.

A year and a half later, I was interviewed by Anne Armstrong Gibson in her crowded Provençal-style kitchen. She looked much older than she had on our previous encounters, as her thin wisps of graying hair were unimpeded by the usual hat. Sitting on a sunny ledge in the company of her boxer dog, two Scottish terriers, and three tabby cats, she unrolled before me a plan for restructuring the Wellspring board of trustees, professional advisory committee, and staff. We discussed the vision for

Wellspring, new directions, and internal issues. Then she looked at me and laughingly said, "Well, tell me about yourself. I'd forgotten who's doing the interviewing here."

I rattled off my credentials: psychologist, psychotherapist, work with children and families, training workshops, specialty in bereavement. I did not think Anne would be particularly impressed by this information. I knew she was looking for someone who could be accountable to her and her team of consultants, someone who could take charge in her absence.

"Well, do you think you can do this?" she asked directly. "I want someone who can get the programs up and running, someone who can take control and initiative and act independently."

I stared at the copper pot on the stove, mixing bowls and tangerines on the countertop, apple peels and chocolate shavings on the linoleum tile. I inhaled deeply, feeling Anne's eyes focused on my face. "I will give it my best," I said. "I'd love the opportunity to try."

"Well then, I'll set you up an interview with Dr. Sutcliffe, the chairman of the advisory board. Of course, you know Simon. If you and he can settle things, then we'll draft up a contract."

I began three weeks later, with no contract, no preliminary orientation, no overlap with my predecessor. A new position had been born and I was to learn by trial and error.

On my second day, a news reporter from the Toronto *Star* came to do a piece on Wellspring. Today I look at the photograph of three staff people, a volunteer, and two cancer patients. I stare at the woman in the black woolen dress, squeezed between a patient and the volunteer, smiling awkwardly at the camera. I know that day marked the beginning of my journey into a new world.

• • •

She looked like a wild woman with her long, frizzy hair throwing itself about in all directions, her baggy, ripped sweatpants, and her oversized sweatshirt with "True Blue" in maroon across the back. *Medusa,* I thought to myself.

"Hi, I'm Amira," she introduced herself in a thick accent, which I identified as Hebrew.

"Hello. Mavis," I responded, as I disentangled myself from gloves, scarf, overcoat, and boots by the front door.

"You must be the new program director. Uh-huh, must be," she muttered, as if talking to herself — or to some invisible presence.

"Sorry, I didn't quite hear you," I lied, as I straightened up. "I'm Mavis, Mavis Himes. First day here, so I'm a bit disoriented."

"I can see that," she said.

"Israeli, right?" I asked, and said a few words in Hebrew.

Amira's eyes lit up. "I'm impressed," she said. She moved in half-time — no sharp motions, but like an elastic band, stretching her muscles in the full range of motion. Her arms and legs moved easily, freely, as if disconnected from her torso, random and loose. When she spoke, she bobbed her head from side to side, causing the masses of curls to shake. Masses of red — auburn red, copper red.

"So, what are you planning to change here?" she asked in a confrontational tone at our second meeting, a week later. "We hear you're on a mission of some sort — a fix-it mission. It was fine the way it was, you know. Everything was just fine, so we really don't need any changes."

"Well, I think I'll just take some time to familiarize myself with the place, get to know some people, like yourself. No big cleanup is about to happen. It does sound as though everyone is upset about Bill leaving. I've heard he had a special way with the members and staff." As I said this, I began to wonder if I *could* fill his shoes. I knew how well Bill had been liked.

Amira hedged; she sniffed out information. She wrinkled her freckled nose as she asked oblique questions and then attacked with her own dogmatic opinions. "What about a staff retreat? Do you think we can expand in some new directions? I was wondering what you felt about some of the new energy-work coming out? You think that stuff is flaky or for real?"

I admired her honesty. I was drawn to her energy. Yet I always felt watched by her, under scrutiny. In return, my eyes would follow as her rounded, fleshy body moved along the corridor past my office.

Amira was one of the two massage therapists at Wellspring. She once told me that all she cared about was the members. "I'm here to help these people whose bodies have been bruised and battered from surgery, chemo, and radiation. That's all I can do here."

Amira was volunteering her time to anoint the bodies of the cancer patients and their caretakers. The members loved her and described her as the woman with golden hands. She was modest with her clients, greeting them by the entrance with a broad smile that exposed the wide gap between her two front teeth.

"Hi, Shirley, come on in. So good to see you again this week." Shirley would reach out to embrace Amira as if she wished she could collapse into her arms.

After a few weeks of testing and probing me, Amira asked if I would like a massage. "The program director looks tired, even a bit fraggled . . . What's that English word? Flustered?"

"Yes, Amira, tired and flustered. I'd love a massage," I replied and like any other member, I followed her down the corridor to the B. B. Bargoon Room, our makeshift massage area.

I felt self-conscious undressing in the sparsely furnished room, which was decorated with donated fabrics in blues and oranges. Shivering in the harsh overhead light, I quickly hid under the covers. Amira knocked on the door and entered the room. She began kneading my shoulders.

"Man, are you ever tense! You need a *lot* of work. I think you need more than one treatment. What do they do in those meetings?"

And then silence, except for ocean sounds from the tape player. I let Amira take over. Her fingers and hands felt powerful, masculine. She adjusted her touch to match the rhythms of my body and gave me just what I needed in order to relax. Even so, I stiffened every once in a while as I momentarily became aware of my vulnerability.

Amira left Wellspring a year after I arrived. I never learned why she left, but I always wondered whether the toll of working with the population at Wellspring became too much for her. I was well aware that burnout was a problem among professionals working in oncology and palliative care. It could often lead to indifference, fatigue, or early retirement to another field.

• • •

Wellspring is a microcosm, a healing community amid the downtown cultural maze of Toronto. Beyond the green-and-white awning and the black shutters, life pulsates. Around the corner on Church Street, men in black leather and heavy neck chains boldly announce their sexual preference. A man in a yellow hard hat leans toward a tall woman whose foot is elegantly poised on his shoeshine stand. In the mouth of the alleyway beside him, a young girl in cut-off red gloves holds out a tin cup, pawing the air like a stray dog. Men in suits are eclipsed by the brash airs of gay couples. Voices vie for attention on the steps of the Second Cup coffee shop. Red pomegranate seeds and date pits litter the sidewalk. Life does not stand still.

Inside the white brick walls of Wellspring, women unbutton coats and sweaters in slow motion and help themselves to Red Zinger tea or a glass of spring water. Men saunter in, timidly at first, unsure whether their presence will be noticed among the predominance of women. In spite of the varied collage of headgear and fashion, light-skinned blondes and dark-skinned brunettes, the thwarted energy of the young and the shuffle of the old, there exists a bond — palpable, kinetic. The common denominator is the lesion — the tumor, the glioblastoma multiforme, the large-cell carcinoma, the fibrosarcoma, the primitive neuroectodermal tumor, the dermatofibrosarcoma protuberans, the endodermal sinus tumor, the dysgerminoma, the immature teratoma — the altered gene that transmits the wrong message, that begins to grow rapidly and multiplies again and again, until it forms a malignant growth. Cancer. The Big C.

Today I arrive early at Wellspring for my weekly group meeting. Aerosol cans, used condoms, gum wrappers, and tissues litter the sidewalk as I approach the paved driveway that welcomes members, volunteers, guests, and trustees. I notice a chip in the black paint of the door; I must remember to mention this to Marny, the office coordinator. The smell of paint and the debris of cigarette butts from the adjacent building swirl in the wind outside the entrance. I take a deep breath before I enter, then pause. I wonder who will have been admitted to the hospital or who may have received bad test results.

My concerns unvoiced, I am greeted by Jane, a petite Australian woman who crushes me with a big bear hug. "It's been a long time! How's the gal?" Jane nearly sweeps me off my feet.

"Wonderful to see you, Jane. You've been home. How was it?" I ask.

"Oh, you know, the folks are still worrying about their young one," and she breaks into laughter. "Look at me — no young chicken! But I've got my hair, though." Jane pulls off her wig, fluffing the peppered salt-and-pepper curls that cap her head.

"Great, Jane. Another few weeks and you'll be able to go out *au naturel*. Any cancellations for the group this morning?"

"No, no one's called so far," Jane answers, checking the board.

Wellspring is a breathing life-space. It sighs and heaves with the voices of its members. I enter the living room and my pulse slows down. The low lighting acts as a sedative. Splashes of pastel blue and deep burgundy accentuate the muted beiges. Palm trees and a creeping philododendron hint at nature's life force.

Preeya is sitting in a corner of the loveseat, her thin legs wrapped in a throw. She greets me quietly, her voice weak from radiation to the vocal cords. I walk over and give her a gentle hug. Preeya still does not know where her primary cancer site is. Her doctors are working in a void.

Within minutes, Carole arrives, tossing down a bag of books to share with the group. I glance at the titles as she serves them up on the coffee table: *Why People Don't Heal and How They Can*, *The Healing Secrets of the Ages*, and *A Cancer Battle Plan*. Carole is struggling with bone pain. She draws me aside and confides that she is worried about Preeya. Then she talks about herself. "I cannot die," she states. "No one dies of cancer in the bones, even if it has metastasized from the breast. You know, it has to spread to a vital organ first."

Carole was diagnosed with breast cancer fifteen years ago. When she first introduced herself to the group, she said she considered herself lucky. "I outlived that doctor's prognosis. Six months he gave me. Can you imagine? What the hell did he know about the will to live? I switched doctors after that."

Carole looks tired today. Her back is stooped. Preeya asks if she got a lift with her husband.

"Yes, I did, but I had a rough night. Not much sleep with the pain. I've called my oncologist, because I feel a new pain in the pelvic area." She lowers herself into the wingback chair and, turning slowly to face me, asks, "How are you, Mavis?"

"Fine," I reply. "I'm doing just fine."

I am the odd one out in this group of women with metastatic cancer. They know that I have never had cancer myself. But they also know that my family history of breast cancer has pushed me toward this work. They know I am prepared to listen without condescension to their concerns. They know I will neither judge their choices nor try to minimize their fears. They know I will not offer false hope, but will help them reach their own conclusions. In return, they will not judge me or demand answers from me.

Lily arrives next. She is dressed smartly in a navy pantsuit, matching navy shoes, and crisply ironed beige shirt. "Good morning. I've just got off the phone with my doctor — I mean, before I left this morning — and good news! My tumor has not grown! It hasn't shrunk either, but no growth is good enough for me."

Still breathless from excitement, she embraces each of us in turn. Wellspring is a family that grieves when it loses a member. Little do we know that Lily will be the first of this group to die — in only six months, from metastasized breast cancer.

The hum of informal chitchat rises as we wait for the fourth member of the group to arrive. Then Tove shuffles across the room, smiling. She looks overwhelmed by her heavy corduroy pants and sunny yellow turtleneck. "Sorry, I'm late. There was a slow-up on the subway."

I look at the loose-fitting clothes and tiny wrists. I think of a puppy that has yet to grow into its skin. I wonder how Tove has the energy to travel by subway. She has been diagnosed with adenocarcinoma, a type of pancreatic cancer, which has metastasized to the liver. Tove defies the profile of high risk — she is under forty, has never smoked, has had no exposure to chemicals, and has never suffered from inflammation of the pancreas. Prognosis: treatable, but not curable.

Tove defies the odds in other ways. She has chosen to forgo palliative chemotherapy, radiation therapy, and adjuvant therapy. She has traveled daily by bus to St. Catharines, almost two hours away, to receive ozone therapy and chelation, and follows a strict macrobiotic diet. This wisp of a woman is also studying homeopathy. She is piloting her own personal study on the will to live, the refusal to give up.

I call the group to order. It is Week Six of a twelve-week group for people with metastatic cancer. "I guess we'll begin now," I say.

Everyone allows her eyes to close and rests her hands, palms up, comfortably on her lap.

"Okay then, just begin to settle in your chair and turn your attention inwards . . ." The words flow easily from my mouth as I too relax my body, eyes closed, palms resting gently on my thighs, feet planted firmly on the burgundy rug. I can hear the breathing of the group members, some irregular, some steady. ". . . Now take some deep breaths and try to gradually lengthen your breathing . . ."

• • •

The first groups I facilitated at Wellspring were general groups that provided eight weeks of support for men and women with varying diagnoses and prognoses, at varying stages of treatment, of varying ages and heights and widths. There were men and women with black hair and blonde hair and no hair, with felt hats and baseball caps, woolen toques and silk scarves. Women with distended bellies and with flat stomachs, with one breast or two breasts or no breasts. Women with makeup and pearls, women with blushed cheeks and diamond rings, women in jeans, in black tights, in woolen skirts, in shorts.

These men and women had walkers, no walkers, canes, no canes, wheelchairs, limps, or no distinguishing gait. They sat in hard chairs or on soft sofas, spoke in rapid, repeated phrases or whispered haltingly, clutched handfuls of tissues, cried and laughed at life's injustices.

The women resembled my mother, my sister, my aunts, my public school teachers, my piano instructor, my best friend's sister, my grandmother. They carved wooden sculptures and painted miniatures on eggshells, they taught and they danced. There were women with children and childless women, women who hugged me at the end of each session, women who shook my hand, and women who simply walked away in sorrow.

Every time I introduced myself as a professional and not a cancer survivor, I searched the room for acceptance. In those initial groups, I was the enemy. More than once I was accused of being an outsider.

"Only if you've had a diagnosis can you *really* understand."

"It's a club, a very special club."

I began to dream about membership in a club that promised no reward, only uncertainty and fear and death. To enhance my confidence, I hid behind the principles of group psychodynamics. According to Irvin Yalom, an authority on group therapy,

> . . . Natural lines of cleavage divide the therapeutic experience into eleven primary factors: instillation of hope, universality, imparting of information, altruism, the corrective recapitulation of the primary family group, development of socializing techniques, imitative behavior, interpersonal learning, group cohesiveness, catharsis, existential factors.

Instillation of hope. Did I really believe in myself and in the efficacy of the group? Did I have the conviction that I could offer hope or help? Did the principles of group psychotherapy apply in the personal search for meaning, for redemption? Could I count on the group for a cathartic experience? Was a "corrective recapitulation" what was needed?

I decided to familiarize myself with the vocabulary of cancer. I studied the *Dictionary of Cancer Words* published by the Canadian Cancer Society: *carcinoma, carcinoembryonic antigen (CEA), CT scan, debulking, familial polyposis, MRI, lymphedema, portacath, Hickman line, thrombocytopenia.*

I became acquainted with the anticancer drugs, their code names, and their side effects: epirubicin, bleomycin, dexamethasone, tamoxifen, melphalan, vinblastine, Taxotere, leucovorin — the ingredients for the chemical cocktails that were ingested or injected daily, weekly, monthly, or bimonthly.

I searched the Wellspring library for books, tapes, and journals, only to enter a new world of alternative medicine, coping techniques, and healing gurus: Bernie Siegel, the Simontons, Lawrence LeShan, Caroline Myss, Dr. Susan Love, Stephen Levine, Dr. Alastair Cunningham. A cornucopia of nutrition guidelines, holistic approaches. A proliferation of red, green, blue, and white volumes, some slim, some bloated with resources and references, some factual, others inspirational, anecdotal.

I borrowed visualization tapes and practiced deep muscle relaxation, tranquility exercises, mindful meditation. I walked the streets of Toronto imagining what it was like to receive a death sentence.

None of this prepared me for the impact of eight men and women complaining about the inhumanity of the medical system, the insensitivity of physicians and technicians, the disfigurement caused by treatments, the gradual erosion of human dignity.

"I found a lump on my breast the size of an orange. I waited a few days and then called my doctor, who felt it and immediately sent me for a mammogram. The results came back negative. My family physician said not to worry. Three months later, I complained again. This thing was growing; it was closer to a grapefruit now. So my doctor scheduled another mammogram. Again the test results came back negative. Then I had an ultrasound: negative. It was only when another tumor popped out, in my other breast, that anything showed up on the tests, and I was admitted to hospital the same day. Diagnosis: metastatic breast cancer. It's hard for me to trust physicians now."

Another voice: "My doctor put me through all the tests when my glands were swollen. He told me I had a virus and gave me Tylenol. Several months later, I learned I had metastatic liver cancer. No one could believe it. My doctor practically avoided me, he was so embarrassed. He had assured me it was nothing."

And another: "I got informed of my diagnosis in the corridor of the hospital. I swear my doctor was just going to take a leak. What was it to him? I wonder how he would have handled it if it was his wife or sister he was informing."

A woman with calico cats appliquéd across her sweatshirt spoke up. "I'm angry, all right. I'm so angry I could burst. But there's one thing I know for damn sure. I don't want to die from fear of my diagnosis, from the medical system failing me, from rage at my family and friends for not supporting me. If I'm gonna die, then godammit, I'm gonna die from my cancer and nothing else. So I've started putting my energy elsewhere."

I sat numbly, inhaling the tension in the room. Words escaped me; my thoughts were frozen. There were many days like that in those first few months when my good intentions were trammeled and my ideas challenged by group revolt. Some days I would leave the group worrying about minor infractions of my own body — the blemish, the nagging pain, the subcutaneous bump — the imagined microscopic cancer cell that could be traveling through me, undetected and unannounced.

"Counter-transference" is a term borrowed from psychoanalytic theory to refer to responses and reactions of the therapist/ analyst that are liable to affect the treatment process. Initially it was a very narrow term, restricted to the definition "all the unconscious processes brought about in an analysis." Today, *counter-transference* is loosely used to refer to all the interfering factors that a therapist carries over from his or her past, both conscious and unconscious, plus all the beliefs he or she holds that may interfere with the therapeutic process.

One day, a woman described how her breast cancer had developed from a calcification in her left breast. My ears burned, my heart began racing. Calcification. I was familiar with that term from my own mammogram results. For a few moments, I could not hear what she was saying, but I managed to force my attention back to the room. When the group was over, I rushed to my office to look it up in *Dr. Susan Love's Breast Book*. I was relieved to learn that only a small percentage of micro-calcifications (small specks of calcium that appear on mammograms) develop into cancer. Eighty percent of these calcifications have nothing to do with cancer, but result from normal wear and tear on the breast or from the natural breakup of calcium that leaves the bones to appear in other places. For the other twenty percent, these potentially precancerous specks can be monitored with regular mammograms, and even when they do develop into cancer, it can take ten years.

3

I was named after my maternal grandmother's sister, Malkah, who was killed in a car accident at the age of fifty. In 1900, as a new bride, she brought my grandmother, then in her early twenties, over to Canada from the Austro-Hungarian Empire to join her and her husband. According to family mythology, Malkah soon after began to resent my grandmother's presence, and quickly arranged a marriage for her.

My maternal grandfather, Hymie Rabinovitch, had worked on the railway lines of Argentina after crossing the Atlantic from Russia at the turn of the century. A quiet man with a wide smile and soft eyes, Hymie moved to northern Quebec a few years after his marriage in order to join his two brothers. He eventually settled in Senneterre, where he owned a store that faced the train station and bore a sign that read "Camille H. Rabinovitch, Prop. General Dry Goods Store." There he traded linens, towels, and clothing in exchange for furs from the Natives.

I look at a picture of my mother as a young girl, smiling coquettishly at the camera as she pats a scraggly dog; two Native boys look on intently. The back of the photograph reads "Mother with mongrel dog Blacky and two Indians." My grandmother made the three-day trek up north once a year in the summertime. My grandfather moved back to Montreal only after my mother married in 1945.

My grandmother, abandoned in her apartment, formed a tightly knit unit with her daughter, my mother. When she was a young child, my mother's health was precarious. Her youthful body fought against scarlet fever, pneumonia, chicken pox, measles, and a number of skin allergies and rashes. Later, the compact duo reversed roles, when my mother had to tend to her mother's failing health.

My grandmother was first diagnosed with breast cancer in her fifties. Only five years separated her two bouts of cancer, and in both cases she had a radical mastectomy, which was the treatment of choice (or no choice) at the time.

My grandmother was a large and buxom woman. I knew that she stuffed her corset with padding before putting on her beige slip and dress. I thought all old people had sagging breasts and therefore wore padded underwear. However, I was puzzled about the size of my grandmother's arms. One day, I screwed up the courage to ask my mother, "How come Bubbe has one fat arm and one skinny arm? How come they're not the same?"

"It's because of an operation she had many years ago," my

mother replied. Only later did I learn that the "fat" arm was the result of having her lymph nodes removed during her second mastectomy. Only when I began working at Wellspring did I learn the name for this condition: lymphedema.

My grandfather died of leukemia at the age of sixty-five. I was completely shielded from his illness and death. When he died, the mirrors were draped with sheets and my mother wore black for a week, while people came and went bringing cakes and casseroles.

Gradually my grandmother began to spend more and more time at our house, until my mother got tired of traveling back and forth between the apartment on Linton Avenue and the house on Queen Mary Road. One day, my grandmother moved into the guest room downstairs for good and I no longer needed to sacrifice my pillow for my Bubbe's sleepovers.

My father said nothing. After all, my grandmother's life had been troubled and unhappy. And besides, what was an only child to do? I was nine years old when my grandmother's furniture was sold, all except her grandfather clock, which was placed in the hallway on our second floor.

My grandmother, unlike many older women today, really looked like a bubbe. Her thin gray hair was cut short and stuck out randomly in all directions, even after it was shampooed. Her skin, fleshy and marbled with veins on her cheeks, was wrinkled and resembled parchment that I had seen at the museum. In her crocheted slippers and pastel shifts, gifts from my mother's travels to the United States, she would pad around the house like a wandering spirit. At times she would watch television in the family room, applauding the contestants on her favorite show, *Let's Make a Deal*. Mostly she would be in her room, resting or sleeping.

On special celebrations, like Mother's Day or birthdays, my grandmother would join the family for a meal at Ruby Foo's or Moishe's. Then she would put on one of the special outfits she had kept from her life with my grandfather. This was typically a black or navy crepe dress under which she wore an enormous corset that would be hooked up by my mother; Linda and I counted forty hooks from hip to chest on each side. Then she would insist on matching, open-toed shoes and crocheted gloves. In her hand she would clutch a small evening bag with a band of rhinestones that my sister and I had once used for playing dress-up.

The final touch would be a dab of red lipstick, which my mother would apply with gentle up-and-down strokes. "Ma, look how nice you look. Now just squeeze your lips together," she would say, beaming. "Just look how nice your grandmother looks," she would repeat to Linda and me.

My grandmother always insisted that she was a subject of the Austro-Hungarian Empire, fondly praising the monarchy of Franz Josef. "He was good for the Jews," she would repeat whenever his name was mentioned. Her devotion to royalty extended beyond the boundaries of her country of origin. She would listen intently to any news about Queen Elizabeth II and would rush to view her glamorous heroine whenever she appeared on television. She also liked to look at photograph books of Euro-pean monarchs. The grandest compliment from her was that you looked more beautiful than the Queen, a statement usually reserved for my mother.

Until the day she died, my Bubbe's dialect was a mixture of English, Yiddish, and German. As a result, I learned to navigate the nuances of two household languages, English with my parents and Yiddish with my grandmother.

My grandmother maintained a strict adherence to Jewish orthodoxy, at least as it pertained to domestic matters. There were two sets of china, a floral set for dairy dishes and a white set with a turquoise rim for meat dishes. Only kosher cuts of meat bought exclusively from a Jewish butcher were allowed into the house. Most of the food we ate was a combination of Old World delicacies (gefilte fish, chopped liver, pickled herring, potato knishes) and "Canadian" specialties (tuna-cheddar melts, spaghetti and meatballs, wieners and beans). It was also my grandmother who insisted on the sanctity of the Sabbath evening meal — lighting candles, breaking the sweet, braided challah, and blessing the fruit of the vine — all of which instilled in me a lifelong nostalgia for ritual and tradition.

In the early years of her residence at our house, I would read to my grandmother from a large volume entitled *An Anthology of Jewish Folktales from Around the World*. My grandmother had her favorites; she would laugh until tears streamed down her cheeks as Moishe accidentally clubbed the baker Meir Lev in the foot, bruising both his toe and his pride. While I also had my favorite stories, she insisted that I reread the same five chapters over and over again.

My grandmother's simple life seemed to revolve around my mother, and thereby indirectly around my sister and me. A simple woman with common sense and a strong spirit, she combined forces with my mother regarding the daily affairs of the house, including meal plans and curfews and discipline for us children.

*

I remember the rituals of cleanliness. As I pass by the bathroom door, I glimpse the image of two women. My mother is helping my grandmother wash. Her back is straight and firm as she kneels over the bathtub rim. My grandmother reclines against the green porcelain of the tub, its smallness accentuating her large form — an elephant in a matchbox.

"Is that you, Mavis?" my mother calls out. "Could you please get me some Epsom salts? There's a box in the laundry room, under the sink."

A dutiful daughter, I retrieve the box and enter the steamy room. I feel like an intruder at some female ritual. I am shy looking at my grandmother's naked body. Folds of flesh roll across her abdomen, shapeless and inert. I notice a few hairs sprouting at the top of her legs. Veins zigzag across her body.

My mother reaches out for the blue-and-white box and pours some crystals into the water. She murmurs some words in Yiddish and English, the dual tongues of the household. I kneel by my mother's side and ask if there is anything else I can do. Suddenly my grandmother slips in the tub, and her arms thrash about. My mother and I reach for her, and gently we readjust her position.

My grandmother's silvery hair is arranged in a bun. My mother pushes a loose strand behind her ear. "Your grandmother has such lovely skin, you know," she reminds me once again. And in the calmness of the afternoon light, I see my grandmother's youthful skin in contrast with the bulk and burden of her aged body. The mastectomies have left her with gaping cavities in her flesh. I think of the framed photograph of my grandfather standing beside my grandmother, a Rubenesque figure in a long print dress.

My mother motions for me to leave. I close the door on the two women, protecting their privacy.

Water rituals. Women and bathing. An image of the mikveh floats up into my consciousness — the ancient water ritual of Jewish men and women. Physically, the mikveh is a small pool of "living water" that is made up in part of rainwater or water from a natural source. Traditionally, those ready to change their existential status — such as by conversion to Judaism or by marriage — go to mikveh to mark that shift. In the Orthodox community, the mikveh is used by married women after menstruation, as well as by men before Shabbat, as a ritual of purification. Physical cleansing, not only in the mikveh, is associated with spiritual cleansing.

Water. Our bodies are two-thirds water. Water is the symbol of birth, of life and creation. As women, water belongs to us; it is the fluid of our bodies, along with blood, the other symbol of life (and death). Water is a connection to Mother Earth. To be reborn is to enter the waters of the womb once more.

• • •

Cancers occurring in animals do not endanger humans.

— American Cancer Society

On Saturday, my friend Ninna and I went to Kensington Market. I was preparing for a dinner party and Ninna had said, "Why don't we spend the morning in the Old World market? We can both do our food shopping together."

Kensington Market is an enclave of bakeries, cafés, vegetable stalls, and poultry shops hidden off Spadina Avenue. I wait for

Ninna at the bustling corner of Baldwin and Augusta. A slim woman hugging an infant and a shopping bag brushes by and knocks me off balance. She mumbles something in an Oriental language. The exotic smells of food permeate the streets. This is a neighborhood of commerce: stalls of leafy greens and peppers, bins of dried currants and legumes, poultry butchers and tantalizing bakeries, fish markets and second-hand clothes. Old World fashion in a New World style.

Ninna waves as she approaches. "Hi, Mave. Sorry, I'm late," she says breathlessly as we embrace. "I couldn't find a parking spot, so I ended up in front of Gwartzman's. A man was just pulling out with a carload of art supplies."

Ninna indoctrinated me into the world of Kensington twenty-five years earlier. There was a ritual to be learned and memorized. Perlmutter's for bagels and knishes; Kaplan's for cheese; the Portuguese grocer for fruit — but check the Israeli on the corner in case the prices are better, although the quality sometimes suffers; the butcher with the green-and-red lettering on the window for poultry; and the Polish meat market for salami, kolbassa, and smoked meat.

Today the colors of the shops have changed. The Hebrew lettering has all but disappeared. Eastern European faces have been replaced by Asian ones. The guttural sounds of Yiddish are still whispered in the back alleys, but the high-pitched vocals of Oriental dialects resound on the main shopping thoroughfare.

Ninna and I make our way down Baldwin Street, brushing past young couples holding hands and chewing on sunflower seeds, peanuts, roasted chestnuts. The streets are slushy and we slide on freshly fallen snow. We hover over tomatoes and oranges, melons and cucumbers. We squeeze and weigh, evaluate and assess the fresh merchandise, choosing only the best.

"You know what Bonnie Stern says about produce selection?" I ask Ninna.

"No, what good advice does the cooking queen have to give?"

"In order to prepare the best dishes, one must begin with the best ingredients. No cheating in that department."

"But of course," Ninna drawls in an exaggerated manner.

We continue on to the Indian shop of dried spices and herbs, the new bakery, and the meat market. I insist on checking out the stores selling Hawaiian shirts and retro fifties and sixties clothing.

"Hey, Ninna, how about this one?" I chuckle, wrapping myself in a chartreuse faux-fur boa.

"I'd say very chic. You might wear it tonight at your dinner party." We both laugh and work our way around the counter of assorted jewelry before leaving.

As we go back outside, Ninna says, "How about a spicy falafel sandwich? I'm famished."

"Good idea. So am I."

We turn into the Baraca Hut and order falafel-in-a-pita sandwiches with all the trimmings: hot sauce, fried eggplant, tomatoes, and lettuce. Fingers dripping with tahini and harissa, we sink our teeth into the soft bread.

"Sid is going for his tests this week," Ninna says as we wait for our coffee. "I'm so nervous that I haven't been able to get a good night's sleep for days now. The incision on his scalp hasn't healed well. It's oozing, and I keep having to replace the dressing. You know, they reassured us at the time that the biopsy was negative. I'm scared, Mave."

I squeeze her arm. "The hardest part is waiting, Ninna," I say, trying to be reassuring. "What time is your appointment? Do you want me to come with you and Sid and wait?"

"It's okay, Mave. Thanks for the offer."

"But call me as soon as you get the results. Promise?" Ninna nods her consent.

A burst of fresh air tickles my nostrils as we go outside. Ninna points a sticky finger down the street and says that she wants to go to the poultry shop next. "The one in the middle of the block. Kosher, like your grandmother would approve of," she sings in her Danish rendition of a Yiddish accent.

In the poultry shop, we are met by a small man carrying cartons of eggs piled up to his hairy nostrils. The smell is familiar — the aroma of Friday night meals: Shabbat candles, white tablecloths, roast chicken, gefilte fish, and tzimmes.

Every Friday night my mother would light the Shabbat candles. I always knew when we gathered around the table that the furniture had been dusted and the carpets vacuumed. I knew that a chicken decked with roasted carrots or delicate parsnip sticks was browning alongside the potato kugel in the oven, and that there would be honey cake for dessert.

My mother would have on a freshly ironed blouse, and over it she wore a special Shabbat apron, a white apron with red and green roses trimming the edges and the pocket. She would stand ceremonially in front of the brass candlesticks on the brass plate given to her by my Aunt Betty. With an expression of quiet dignity, she would place a tea towel on her head, strike a match, and light the candles, then close her eyes and move her hands above the flames, murmuring as if in some magical relationship with a force ignited by the burning candles. As a young child, I would stand straight as a sentinel, mesmerized by the impact of a power I could not name.

Ninna places her order: two large capons and three small roasting chickens. "Please clean them well. No feathers, thank you. And I'll have the giblets on the side."

"What about the feet, lady? You want them left on for soup?" asks a voice from the back.

"No, thanks," Ninna calls out into the vapors of the shop.

"Ninna, that's the secret ingredient of chicken soup. Don't you know?" I whisper in her ear.

"What, you think I'm Jewish or something?" she jokes, chiding me in her Yiddish accent.

"Okay, okay. Don't say I haven't tried to teach you a thing or two," I laughingly respond. We leave with three more plastic bags, which Ninna carefully packs into her shopping basket.

Ninna has finished with her purchases and so have I. We weave our way through the cluttered streets back to the car and once again hug each other goodbye.

"Now, don't forget to call after the doctor's appointment," I remind Ninna. "I'll be thinking of you."

"And don't forget to give my love to Lawlor."

Twenty-five years before I discovered the maze of Toronto's Kensington Market with my friend Ninna, I accompanied my grandmother to the Rachel Street market in Montreal.

My grandmother is wearing support stockings and thick-soled black shoes with open toes. In her left hand she carries a cloth shopping bag with wooden handles. She walks quickly, using her cane recklessly, and beckons me to follow. I trail behind her, my eyes glued to the pavement, until she stops at a narrow stall heaped with sawdust. She motions to a man in a bloodstained apron and points her cane to a crate hedged by two empty cages.

"That one in there. That one. I want to see that one," she says, tapping the crate lightly.

I peer inquisitively through the slats; my gaze is met by a dark eye staring back at me. The man in the apron slowly opens the crate and pulls out a squawking chicken.

"A finer one, a gut one," he says, proudly displaying his screeching specimen.

"How much? How much?" my grandmother repeats.

There is a quick exchange of more words and money. The man disappears into the back of the stall, only to reappear with a bundle wrapped in newspaper, which he drops into my grandmother's shopping bag. We leave and move on.

To kosher a chicken not only means that it has been slaughtered with the least amount of bloodletting, but also that it has been cleaned and purified according to strict rituals. Upon our return home, my grandmother would pluck the feathers, including those trapped in the folds of skin, and run cold water from the tap over the fowl for fifteen minutes. Then it would be salted and left to sit on a wooden board to drain for another thirty minutes. Finally, it would be ready for cooking. I only remember seeing a heap of dismembered life.

"You must remove all the blood, all the impurities, *mein kind*," she would say as she indoctrinated me into the world of Jewish dietary laws. For women only.

• • •

The room is stuffy today. I have not seen this group since the end of June. The graduate metastatic group, an ongoing support group, is reconvening for the first time after the summer break. There is an animated energy in the room.

Pat says, "I find it so difficult to go to my aquafit classes. The gym has open change rooms and I hide in a corner, facing the lockers and trying to squeeze into my bathing suit as fast as I can. Then when I'm done the class, I try to wrap this big body into a towel the size of a postage stamp. It's not me, it's the others I want to protect. It's like I'm trying to prevent others from feeling uncomfortable on my behalf."

"I know exactly what you mean," chimes in Liz. "I feel so ugly, so mutilated. Even my best friend couldn't look when I tried to show her my scar."

"It's just that I feel like some kind of freak. They want to look, I know it. I feel their eyes, and it makes me want to scream." Pat's eyes fill with tears.

"I can't stand that shit. I tell you, I have no patience for it." Sarah shakes her head of blonde curls as she speaks. "My chest — this is my badge of courage. No way I worry about scaring others. And if I do, well, good for them. This will wake them up. This just gives me so much permission. If others are forced to stare at my scarred breast and it puts things in perspective for them, that's a damn good thing. I refuse to be apologetic to anyone."

A round of applause breaks out. In unison they cheer, "Right on, right on!"

"You know what?" Liz begins again. "I do aquafit with all these seniors. Well, *those* are ugly bodies, no kidding — a bunch of overweight women who make me feel youthful and attractive. And they're not that much older than I am. I try not to focus on my boobs. I do avoid exposure, but I slip into my bathing suit with the falsies and *voilà*, no one needs to know."

"Well, I've had reconstruction but I still feel self-conscious. No kidding. I still have these scars, one boob is still larger than the other, and with this new biopsy, they've messed up my "good" breast. So a lot of good the surgery did," Linda says.

"I know exactly what you mean," Pat offers. "I swear I feel like a bruised potato with all the rotten parts scooped out."

I think about recent media images of women with their mastectomy scars, publicly celebrating an alternative vision of beauty. I see a woman on exhibit in a gallery with a pastoral landscape tattooed across her flattened chest. Aren't these brave women to be congratulated for their efforts to restore a sense of aesthetics and womanliness to their bodies? But in this shaded room I hear the voices of women who continue to feel silenced, flawed, and mutilated by the marks on their bodies.

"I hate to change the topic, but I'm on this antioxidant diet, and the chlorine in the swimming pool is supposed to be toxic. So does anyone else have any information about this?"

• • •

> Cancer can occur at any age, even in the newborn. However, the probability of developing cancer increases with age. This is due to both the natural aging of the body and the length of time the body has been exposed to environmental factors that can cause cancer.
>
> — American Cancer Society

Last night, I dreamed about my mother. She approached me, wrapped in a towel. As she came near, she dropped the towel, exposing one healthy breast and the place where the second breast should have been. A deep diagonal scar sliced her left chest into two unequal parts. I averted my eyes and wanted to run. When I looked again, my mother had disappeared. In her place, I was confronted by several women with pregnant breasts swollen like melons, each woman wrapped tightly in a dress that was splitting open. Moaning sounds erupted across the room. I awoke in a sweat.

I was never able to look at my mother's mastectomy scar, a pinkish-reddish line like a railway track, the flesh scooped out — a flat surface where rounded flesh once swelled. A strange tightening sensation would grip my insides.

I had heard about my mother's diagnosis and surgery from my father. A routine mammogram revealed a lump. A needle biopsy confirmed malignant cells. The doctor did not hesitate to recommend that the entire breast be removed immediately, leaving my mother no choice. Twenty-four hours later, she awoke from the anesthesia a scarred and mutilated woman.

"We had no choice," my father said across the long-distance

wires. "The doctor said it was better not to take any chances. Your mother is in shock."

The words splashed against me, dripping from my shoulders. My world was three hundred and fifty miles away. I could not react. At the time, I had just moved in with my boyfriend and was experimenting with the pleasures of sexual abandon. My breasts were firm and sensual, a source of newly discovered erotic sensations. That night I slept in my boyfriend's arms. In the morning, I booked a flight to Montreal.

My mother wants me to look at her scar again. It is several years after her surgery. "Look, I want you to see this one more time before I have my reconstruction."

I wonder if she senses my discomfort, remembers my initial hesitation, feels offended.

"This is the last time you will see your mother like this," she continues. "No more prostheses, no more falsies, no more . . ." Her voice drops. "You know, your father never minded. He said it was more important that I have my health. He was so supportive." My mother is being unusually talkative. "The doctor told me I am a good candidate for this implant. He says the technology has advanced and there are positive results. If the first procedure works, then he says he may be able to make a nipple as well, from the other tissues."

I listen. I cannot imagine the loss. My mind races with questions that I cannot ask. What if your body rejects the implant? What about the new scars? How safe is this operation? What about the news on the dangers of implants? What if it looks worse? What if . . . ? My mother lifts her sweater and I stare blankly at her chest.

When I return to Toronto, I call a plastic surgeon. He tells me there have been significant advances in breast reconstruction techniques. "The most popular is the TRAM flap, which uses the woman's own tissue to build a breast," he says casually. "Alternatively, there are saline or silicone breast implants."

Becoming more clinical, he proceeds to inform me that women who have undergone reconstructive surgery report a more positive body image, improved self-esteem, and a more satisfying quality of life. "The studies in the journals all claim that women experience a renewed sense of wholeness and balance, of comfort in dress, and in physical relations," he says. "My patients tell me the same thing."

I thank him politely for his time and put down the receiver. I repeat the phrases to myself: "renewed sense of wholeness and balance," "comfort in dress . . . in physical relations." I want to believe it all. But do we really know anything about the unconscious meanings of corrective surgery? Do the phantoms of mutilation and loss of sexual identity continue to haunt these women? Are they really more ready to resume sexual intimacy? Are they more fulfilled as women?

My mother calls me a week later, right after the operation. Her surgery has been successful. She knows it will take a few months for the swelling to settle and the final results to be seen. I never ask her whether she feels more sensual and womanly.

The clothes in my mother's wardrobe smell sweet and floral —

Cabochard by Grès. I like to bury my nose in my mother's sweaters and scarves. Their scent is as exotic as the perfume bottle with the beige velvet bow that sits atop her dresser tray.

When she was younger, my mother loved fashion. Her clothes would be lined up in perfect order in the closet — dresses, skirts, shirts, shoes on the floor, purses on top — ready to wear. While my friends' mothers wore more flamboyant colors, my mother dressed in subdued, tailored clothes for daytime wear: tweed skirts in autumn shades with beige cashmere sweaters, or black knits with softly colored sleeveless tops. She once owned a burnt-orange coat dress that I wanted her to leave me in her will. And then there was the textured gray suit with the metallic buttons that I also secretly coveted.

But it was on Saturday nights, when my mother and father dressed up for special occasions, that my mother's beauty and taste really glowed. I close my eyes and images whirl behind them: my mother, jet-black hair tied back, dressed in a sequined gown or a slinky evening dress; my mother in a beige Balmain gown or a green chiffon dress with double spaghetti straps, flowing to her ankles; my mother, who made me think of an Italian princess or an exotic actress; my mother, who was always so conscious and proud of her appearance.

As a young child, I wished to grow up to emulate my mother's charm and poise. As an adolescent, I resented my mother's youthful appearance and my boyfriends' comments about her. I rebelled against her seeming preoccupation with appearances and cosmetic materialism. Today she is in her mid-seventies, and I admire her still-youthful look and her attractiveness, hoping that I have inherited some of those same genes. Yet I continue to wonder how she feels about her body and how she has coped with all its changes. And I wonder too about my grandmother, how *she* managed to deal with the devastation to her body.

• • •

Women and their bodies. It is hard to imagine a more intimate relationship. In many ways, we are our bodies. They contain the physical manifestation of our psyches. We are born into a body out of which we develop both physically and mentally. Freud postulated that the ego, the part of our psyche that represents reason and common sense, is first and foremost a bodily ego, "a surface entity from which both internal and external perceptions may spring."

According to Jacques Lacan, a French psychoanalyst, the body is the locus of *jouissance*, a paradoxical term that refers to the "painful pleasure" of physical experiences. It is a space in which many instances of *jouissance* circulate. In this schema, the body is a sexual body, the source of sexual urges and passions and the thrust of unconscious libidinal energy.

As always, images of women abound in the pages of fashion and beauty magazines, are flaunted by the cinematographer's lens and taunt the audience, and are fantasized about by men and women alike. Titillating images of women twisting, bending, stretching, arching, in poses of natural and unnatural grace; motion shots of women dressing, bathing, cooking, driving, playing; frozen moments of women laughing, smiling, crying, pouting, screaming.

In the twenty-first century the body is no longer viewed in

religious terms as the vessel of the soul, on loan to us from a divine presence, or a container for spiritual development that is our responsibility to purify, nurture, and safeguard. In today's culture, the body is worshipped and revered simply as an object of beauty and of sexual gratification.

Anna Globus's shop was on Queen Mary Road in Montreal, a second-floor walk-up with creaky floorboards and chipped paint. Anna Globus represented initiation into the world of grown-ups, a rite of passage into womanhood — like menstruation, like shaving, like being able to refer to condoms in everyday speech.

Anna Globus did not sell training bras, and fitness bras had not yet been designed. The brassieres she sold came in size 30AA and went up from there. When I accompanied my sister there for her first fitting, I had been forced to wait in the front lounge. Today it was my turn to enter the realm of the fitting rooms in the back.

Anna, a short woman with a full bust and a tight sequined sweater set, greeted my mother and me. "Is it your first time?" she asked with a smile. When my mother nodded in affirmation, Anna shuffled off in her pink padded slippers and returned with an index card.

"Okay, then," she began, "Name. Address. Date of birth."

After a few moments of written introduction, I was led to a cubicle and told to undress to my waist. Cold hands placed a tape measure under my arms, across my chest and around my back. "Mm-hmm, okay. Mm-hmm," she murmured. Then, abruptly, "Okay, young lady. Let's see what we can find for you today."

My mother told me to stand up straight and not to slouch. Anna Globus returned with five bras draped over her arm like clean laundry. "Let's start with these. Now put your arms through here. That's it," she instructed, as I struggled with the thin cotton straps. "Now I want you to bend over. That's a girl. Okay, and just jiggle yourself into the cups. Okay, now straighten up. Okay, now let's just tighten these straps a bit on the shoulders. Okay, then."

She turned to me, no longer treating me like a mannequin, and asked, "Now, how does that feel?"

Hmmm . . . awful, I thought to myself. I just wanted to run out. I no longer wanted to be a woman. My little breasts were hidden under cotton padding, and I thought I looked goofy. My mother and Anna Globus exchanged words and knowing looks while I got dressed.

After paying the bill at the front desk, my mother handed me a pink paper bag. I took it and turned it so the printed "Anna Globus" lay face down against my leg.

A long, slender mirror hangs behind the door. It is a modest piece of glass that waits like a lonely sentinel until a figure appears in front of it. Then the mirror comes to life with the colors of the human form: satin peach and soft taupe, caramel and antelope, honey pecan and velvet caramel.

In front of the mirror stands a girl with cascading curls. She wants to be a ballerina. She twirls and pirouettes, admiring her image in the length of glass. She waves and the mirror returns her greeting. She performs for the mirror, twirling and swirling. Then her mother's image appears suddenly behind her, a towel draped over her arm. Two silhouettes melt into one as the mother enfolds the girl in the towel.

The girl's name is Claire. "*Claire de lune*," her father croons as he rocks her to sleep. In the future she will learn how the moon's rhythms coincide with the rhythms of her own cycles, and this will bring her comfort. Rhythm, cyclicality — there is harmony between her body and the celestial forces, harmony between her inner self and the great cosmos.

But let us return to the room where a small girl enacts a play, a game of adoration of the image in the mirror. A game in which ballerinas are twirled by handsome princes. Let us suppose that, in precocious anticipation of her own development or, even more likely, in envy of her mother's mature body, she points to the tiny spots on her chest and asks gleefully, "Will my little titties grow big like yours?"

And her mother, with a proud smile, responds, "Well, of course, my dear. Of course they will. You too will be a woman some day."

Thirty-five years later, Claire stands in front of a magnetic resonance imaging machine. The images it records are multi-dimensional. Claire will slide into the machine's metal body; she will not see the images on the screen. But she has seen the pictures from her mammogram: dark "hot spots" indicate the growth of malignant tumors in her left breast.

Today Claire is sitting in a circle of Wellspring members. "My breast is weeping. There is a seeping sore under my shirt. This breast, once voluptuous," she says, cupping her hand over it, "is now oozing with fluids. It makes me sick."

Some of the other women in the room nod their heads. Claire continues, "I knew something was wrong. I felt a lump in my breast the size of a ping-pong ball. No, the size of a golf ball. Then it became the size of a tennis ball."

Precision. The details of precision, the precision of measurement. The imprecision of measured responses. The response of the group, in unison, like a Greek chorus:

> *Cancer is subversive. It is the silent enemy.*
> *Cancer is subversive. It is the silent enemy.*
> *Cancer is invisible. It threatens from within.*
> *Cancer is invisible. It threatens from within.*

• • •

The sign at the top of the stairs reads "Breast Imaging Patients." My appointment is for 8:15 a.m. and already a row of women, sitting like mannequins in a store window, lines the gray hospital wall. The sign above the receptionist requests that people kindly have their health insurance number and requisition slip ready. Today the receptionist repeats a new refrain, "Have a seat. The printer is down. I am trying to see whether they will accept handwritten forms upstairs. Please have a seat and be patient."

Women are used to waiting. Not always patiently, but waiting, nevertheless. Waiting nine months for labor pains. Waiting years for sons and husbands to return from battle. Waiting for sons and daughters to return from school and husbands to return from work. Waiting for the stuffed turkey, the marinated meat, the duck *à l'orange*, the pecan pie to emerge from the oven.

Waiting with bated breath, with urgency, with legs apart or legs together, waiting for the results of tests, or simply waiting to pass the time away.

I return to my seat and join the other women slumped in their chairs. The woman beside me is clutching a Toronto *Sun,* a requisition form, a beige trench coat with fur trim, a red scarf, and an overstuffed purse.

"The printer is down," she says. "What did they do in the good old days? They've forgotten how to write is what I think." And she accidentally drops her scarf. As she reaches down, I notice her metallic pink nail polish.

I search my handbag for a piece of paper. As I fumble around, a man appears — handsome, with shoulder-length blond hair and soft blue eyes. He has come to fix the printer, the women whisper in unison. We all stare at the handsome man, or gawk — he is the only male we have seen this morning in the imaging department.

Eventually I am called to the front desk. The woman in the East Indian head-scarf behind the computer does not look up. She simply says, "Follow the yellow line to third-floor reception, Room 373. Elevators on your right." I take the elevator one floor up and follow the yellow line to Room 373. This is my eleventh mammogram. I am an old-timer.

My friend Rhonda says she hates mammograms. She calls it "frying eggs." She says that her breasts are tiny, and it embarrasses her when the technician inevitably comments on the difficulty of X-raying women with small breasts. "I want to apologize for causing them problems," Rhonda admits sheepishly. "Can you believe it?"

The woman facing me in the waiting room is holding a clipboard with a form on it. She asks the volunteer in the blue dress — her name tag says "Marjorie" — what she should do with the form. A balance statement. A balanced statement. I have memorized my responses: name, address, date of birth, date of onset of menstruation, date of last menstrual cycle, date of pregnancy. A personal history followed by a family history — a family history of breast cancer. I tick off all the boxes: grandmother, mother, sister, maternal aunt, paternal aunt.

I try to distract myself by reading the signs. "Are You Taking Tamoxifen?" is looking for volunteers for a study. "Please Note: The Use of Cellular Phones Is Strictly Prohibited." "No Deodorants or Perfume Please." I notice a new sign posted on two of the walls. It is the pink rose that first catches my attention.

> For Best Mammogram Possible: When your mammogram is taken, we will need to compress (flatten) your breasts. Compression is important because it helps ensure:
> - A more even breast thickness, allowing a clearer "picture" to be taken for your doctor to examine.
> - A lower dose of radiation (X-rays).
>
> So please try to relax and let us know if your exam becomes too uncomfortable. We care about you.

Two women are chatting beside me, one with thick makeup and cerulean eyeshadow and the other in black tights and an oversized pullover. Mother-and-daughter bonding. When I was twenty-two, I had no idea what a mammogram was, and I certainly did not know that my mother was sitting in a similar room in a faded green hospital gown, near a sign that said "Please Notify the Technician if You Are Pregnant."

A cheery blonde comes in and addresses the room. "Hi, I'm Linda, the volunteer. Is everyone being looked after?" We all nod in acknowledgment. "The printer is down," she continues.

My name is called. "This way, please," a woman says. I recognize the technician from previous years. Her name tag says "Alice." "This way, across the hall." I am crossing the yellow line.

I immediately strip off my gown in anticipation of the ritual. This year there are new machines, shiny beige-and-black robots with large, pincer-like arms. Alice is gentle, lifting my breast like an expensive cut of meat.

"Now this will feel cold, honey," she says. "I want you to stand over here and I'll just lift your breast a bit higher on the tray. That's it. Now just lean forward a bit more and place your other arm on this rest. Now hold your other breast out of the way."

It is just before my menstrual cycle, and my breasts are swollen and tender. My hormones find their way to my tear ducts. The compression is so strong that I squeal, "Ouch!"

"I'm sorry," Alice says. "These new machines print out a compression reading. It's written right on the film, so they know if we're cheating or not."

Machines designed by men? *Even in the Breast Imaging Department, Big Brother is watching*, I think to myself.

"Now just hold your breath and don't move," Alice continues as she disappears out of sight. "That's a girl." Her voice descends in appreciation. Then she reappears from behind the partition. "Okay, now we'll do the other side." We reverse the position and I try to be as accommodating as possible. Then there is a second set of X-rays before I am told to have a seat back in the waiting room.

Ten minutes later, I am called back for another shot; the radiologist wants a magnification. The previous year when this happened, I had to reschedule a second appointment, so I am relieved to be spared a second trip. This time the procedure is even more acrobatic and painful. Alice tries to be sympathetic; she tells me that she thinks the men who designed these machines forgot that breasts were attached to bodies. We both chuckle.

Once again I return to the waiting room. Alice reappears and tells me that I must reschedule another appointment, for an ultrasound. The mammogram results are ambiguous.

That night, I dream that I have breast cancer. Blood drips from my nipple — big red drops, like rusty water from an old faucet. I wake up screaming. Lawlor immediately wakes up and holds me tightly, rocking me back to sleep.

I return to the hospital two weeks later. I retrace my steps and wait once again in Room 373. Finally I am called in by a technician. As I lie in the dark, she tells me that she is going to apply some gel to my breast and that it will feel cold. I hold my breath. The gel is cold, and gooey. As her left hand gently moves the scanner over the gel, the technician's attention is riveted on a screen showing the tissue of my breast. I am too nervous to watch. After ten minutes, she tells me that I may leave. The procedure is over.

Ten days later, I receive a phone call from my family physician to tell me that the "suspicious-looking" dark area was felt to be nothing significant. I am to reschedule another routine mammogram next year.

• • •

In November 1993 in Montreal, I attended the first Canadian National Forum on Breast Cancer, a convention of oncologists, surgeons, epidemiologists, social workers, psychologists, and nurses, as well as breast cancer patients. This was the first conference that brought together both professionals and cancer patients from across the country. The convention center was filled with hundreds of people roaming the halls and lounges.

Leading authorities on the medical and psychosocial issues of breast cancer addressed such topics as the use of support groups in the healing process, the influence of diet in metastatic disease, and risk factors in the diagnosis of breast cancer. Sharon Batt, president of Breast Cancer Action in Montreal, gave a moving testimony of her own experience with breast cancer. Other breast cancer activists, spurred on by lessons learned from the AIDS community, filled the audiences, asking questions, demanding more research, and questioning the allocation of funds.

Another staff member from Wellspring and I carefully unpacked our public relations material and settled ourselves into a display booth at the forum, handing out brochures and answering questions about Wellspring, cancer, and tourist attractions in Montreal. As I sat in the display corridor, I wrote the following poem in my journal:

AT THE NATIONAL FORUM

As children we snickered. Breasts.
A word of adult grandeur, of dirty connotations.
Or was it the taste of a sexual underground

which caused us to cover our mouths in whispers?
Back-snapping paraphernalia, humiliation.
Little boys laughing uncontrollably at their antics.

Today, women's breasts are on parade.
A celebration of mammary glands, of women's flesh.
Mothers, daughters, sisters, partners, colleagues.
Fighters against a common enemy.
The speakers present their latest findings
A combination of facts and figures,
configurations and confabulations,
Statistics run rampant, diagrams dazzle,
A linguistic maze of tumorigenesis, germ line mutations,
oncogenes.
A male researcher
struts by, his tie a digital analog
Red cherries in tandem.
Or is it, upon closer examination
pairs of bleeding nipples marching down his shirt?

Cancer survivors inspire:
wounded heroes, charred chests,
battling, surviving the warring flesh.
They fight to be heard.
A soprano voice amidst the droning bass of spinning engines
a life-and-death fight to the end:
"Take charge," "Advocate for yourselves," "Wake up to
your priorities."
The men listen, nervously tapping their feet:

"What does this mean? This forum of
women, this accelerating
energy. What if these exploding
hormones were to be unleashed?"

In the display room outside the lecture halls
pictures and posters abound.
TV monitors depicting breasts: pink breasts, peach breasts,
an artist's delight, a palette of different sizes and shapes.
Breasts touched and prodded by antiseptic hands,
dehumanized, sterilized, no passion, no erotic imagery
here. Only a demystification of flesh.

The female delegates walk up and down the aisles.
They speak in muffled voices of the "continuum of care."
Corseted against their bodies, the hidden
Plums of sensuality are kept out of sight.

But then the young woman sashays across the hall,
An innocent bystander, curious, inquisitive about the events
Pendulous flesh languorous beneath her clothes.
She has not been informed of the rules.
The men leer, their tongues wagging
snickering boys
They have forgotten hormone receptors, breast epithelium
cells,
negative growth receptors.
Once again, their manhood rises as they turn to follow
the young

woman with their eyes.
She turns to leave.
Harmony is restored.

Shortly, the speeches will end, the discussion groups disband.
Recommendations on behalf of malignant
breasts will be made.

A number of breast cancer initiatives were started as an outcome of this conference. Discussion and community groups were formed in many remote rural settings. In Ontario, the Breast Cancer Information Network was set up to look at three government-sponsored areas of development: the role of medical practitioners in dealing with cancer patients, the pooling and dissemination of material on breast cancer, and the development of provincial resource centers.

• • •

I enter a room at Sunnybrook Hospital and feel several pairs of eyes turn toward me and stare. I have just arrived half an hour late for a meeting with some senior physicians from the College of Family Practice. It is the first meeting of the Breast Cancer Information Network, and I have been invited as a representative from Wellspring. The meeting is an attempt to establish a dialogue with physicians regarding the educational needs of patients with breast disease.

"Excuse me," I mumble as I slide into an empty chair. I glance quickly at the ten men and two women seated around the boardroom table. The chairwoman acknowledges my arrival with a nod. The man beside me is tapping his pencil on the sheet with the meeting agenda. I notice a blur of doodles on a second sheet of paper.

A man in a gray suit across the table is speaking, waving his hands for emphasis. "I am just wanting to make sure I get this right. You are suggesting that physicians spend *more* time with their patients explaining the differences between non-malignant breast disease and cancer. You think we have the time to sit down and discuss these issues casually? What, over coffee? Do you know how many interest groups like this one have requested more time, more education, more empathy, more —" He stops in mid-sentence, his face red and the veins on his temple pronounced.

"I am sorry," he continues unexpectedly. "We are not psychologists. We are not trained to be hand-holders. We are concerned with the body and that is what we do best. If we were to spend time discussing prevention and education and who knows what else with each of our patients, as you are suggesting, we would never have time for the *real* issues."

"Excuse me," I hear myself say, "but perhaps there is a common thread among all those interest groups you mentioned. Perhaps something is being identified that needs physicians' attention so patients don't run around getting second and third medical opinions because no one explained to them what is going on with their bodies — especially their family physicians, with whom they supposedly have the longest relationship."

"Excuse me, I did not catch your name, Miss . . . ? I don't believe we were introduced," the man in the gray suit says to me.

"It's actually Dr. Himes. I am a psychologist and the program director at Wellspring," I calmly reply.

"Well, Dr. Himes, perhaps this is more your territory then."

The chairwoman intervenes. "Perhaps we need to consider some initiatives, some type of seminar or workshop on patient education, or —"

She is cut off by a man with wavy hair and a white goatee. "Do you know who you are competing with in terms of medical conferences? Aside from the 'softness' of the topic we are discussing, you would be in competition with incentive conferences sponsored by pharmaceutical companies, with bonus ski packages to Utah or Colorado. I don't think you would have any luck there."

"But what about the concept? Are we even agreed that physicians need to develop their communication skills?"

There is general mumbling around the room.

Once again I speak up. "I am wondering whether we should focus our efforts more on medical students who are just coming into the system. Maybe if they are made more aware of the importance of medical communication at the start, it will become part of the routine. Maybe the established physicians are too set in their ways and we should redirect our energy."

I feel the tension in the room. Comments go back and forth without any resolution. The chairwoman tables the subject for the next meeting and urges us to move on to the next item on the agenda. The meeting is finally adjourned after two hours. As I get up to leave, the man in the gray suit introduces himself.

"I did not formally introduce myself. I am Dr. W. I apologize for the misunderstanding."

I raise my voice inquisitively, "Was there a misunderstanding?"

"Well, you seem to have the impression that senior doctors are inflexible and set in their ways. We are not all like that, you know. It's just that we have the experience behind us that leads us to certain conclusions."

"I really must go," I say quickly and dash out.

I am furious. I am raging. I race home, slamming the door behind me. I throw my briefcase on the floor.

"Those stupid assholes! I hate them — all of them! Those goddamn doctors! Where do they get off thinking they're so goddamn holy?"

Lawlor motions for me to sit down. He is used to my occasional theatrical outbursts. "Whoa, slow down," he says in a calm voice.

I collapse into a chair and catch my breath. I wait until the tension in my body subsides. Then I promise myself that, in the morning, I will speak to some medical colleagues about the need for patient education and doctor-patient communication.

4

Cancer is a process whereby a loss of control of normal cell division and multiplication produces a tumour that can invade adjacent tissues and metastasize, that is, implant cancerous cells at a site that is noncontiguous to their origin, where abnormal multiplication continues.

— K. Kiple

My mother's best friend was Lolly Cobrin. Like my mother, Lolly always wore tweed skirts and cashmere sweaters with pearl buttons. Every Passover, she would send my grandmother a dozen pink roses. She loved opera; whenever we visited her house, it was filled with the voice of Maria Callas or Mario Lanza singing in a foreign language. When I was six years old, she initiated me into the world of dance by taking me to a performance of *Coppélia* at the Place des Arts. When I was ten, I learned that Lolly had been diagnosed with ovarian cancer. She died within six months.

But it was when my Aunt Jean (not my real aunt, but a surrogate family member) was diagnosed with breast cancer that I really became familiar with the devastation, both physical and mental, of this disease. Aunt Jean and Uncle Irwin were neighbors when we lived in our first family house. They had two daughters the same ages as my sister and me. We all used to play in the alleyway behind the houses on our street.

When I was in high school and old enough to understand that life could be held in suspension, Aunt Jean was diagnosed with breast cancer. For two years, she was in and out of the hospital for chemotherapy sessions. She would return home sick, vomiting and exhausted. There would be phone calls back and forth between my mother and Uncle Irwin checking on Aunt Jean's flickering life force. My mother tended to be secretive about her friend's progress and never volunteered reports to my sister and me. Instead, she would sigh heavily when talking about "Jeannie's girls" having to witness their mother's illness. In my mind, cancer became a huge monster that attempted to devour one's life from the inside.

As my mother spoke about Aunt Jean in hushed whispers to her friends, I realized there was something taboo about this disease. Cancer was associated with shame and with the stigma of being "different." In my adolescent mind, I knew breasts were not something to be discussed publicly. Breasts were secret and personal. So in addition to my mother's avoidance, I too shied away in discomfort from this mysterious threat called breast cancer.

When I was finally allowed to visit Aunt Jean, I greeted a woman whose haggard face I no longer recognized. It was as if my fears had been confirmed. Only gradually, over many months, did her strength and jocularity return. Yet in my mind there remained a shadow over her. From then on, I was less certain about the reliability of the human body and its functioning.

• • •

Like all parents of young children, my parents wanted to protect my sister and me from bad news. Certain issues were spoken about in Jewish, the "adults only" language of our house. And like all children of dual-language homes, we understood a lot more than our parents realized. After supper, there might be references to my father's heart condition, a test result, a doctor's visit — always in muted tones, as my sister and I supposedly played in the adjacent room. Frozen into inaction, we stretched to listen.

I always knew that cancer was something bad, monstrous, and scary. No one had ever told me; it was something that had infiltrated my repertoire of fears by osmosis.

I remember the first children's group Liz Nichols and I conducted at Wellspring. Six boys and girls, aged seven to ten, sat shyly in a circle on the floor, not knowing what to expect. As we explained the purpose of the group, Steven, an outspoken child whose father had stomach cancer, said, "Oh, you mean it's about my father's dying from cancer. My mom cries a lot, and then when I walk into her room, she pretends she's just blowing her nose."

And Tamara, who had been coloring squiggles on a piece of paper, blurted out, "Oh, yeah, I know what you mean. My parents think I don't know what's been going on. But I hear them talking on the phone, I see my mom's hair falling out, I notice her staying in bed all the time. They seem to think I don't notice. Like I don't notice all the doctor's appointments and hospital visits and going to and from babysitters?"

Like adults, children have a tremendous need to create order out of disorder, to make sense out of nonsense or chaos. Lacking the sophisticated cognitive abilities of their parents, they are more limited in their judgments and must rely on partial facts, fabricating tales and distorting truths to fill in the blanks. Like adults, they resort to their imagination where gaps in logic require connections. The result is often a frightening version of what Mommy or Daddy may be experiencing, or perhaps a fatal prognosis that does not exist.

In the children's group, Liz and I talk about cancer using the metaphor of a garden with flowers and weeds. Like cancer cells, the weeds take over the garden, choking the pretty flowers. Surgery is like weed removal; chemotherapy is like applying chemical pesticides and insecticides to the whole garden; radiation therapy is like direct application of poisons to particular weeds.

Liz and I draw diagrams of cancer cells, bring in medical supplies and chemo dolls, and show demonstrations of various treatments. We write on flip charts:

The body produces good cells.
Sometimes, the body also produces bad cells.
Cancer is a disease in which the bad cells start to take over the good cells.

Cancer cells are stupid.
They don't follow the rules.
So we try to get rid of them.
Some people may die of cancer, but Mommy and Daddy and the doctors are going to do everything they can to make sure they don't die.
We all get scared.
Sometimes we get scared when we don't know what is going to happen.
Mommy will be tired from the treatments and Daddy may be grumpy and worried, so everyone has to help each other to get through this period.

When Steven and Tamara left the first group meeting, they were laughing and discussing what games to bring in the following week. Their mothers looked at me quizzically. I smiled. I knew the children had done their work for the day.

• • •

On a snowy Sunday afternoon, I decide to visit the picture collection at the Toronto Reference Library. The librarian smiles when she hands me the folders labeled "Microscopy," "Pathology," and "Cancer" in which I will look for photo slides of cancer cells.

"You might find something in any of these," she says, adjusting the glasses on the bridge of her Roman nose. "They're really quite beautiful and colorful." Then she adds, "Such a shame that beauty can be so destructive. Reminds me of seeing my uncle's farmhouse burn down when I was a child. I thought it was the most beautiful sight I had ever seen . . . until I woke up the next morning." And she walks off.

As I flip through the pages of intricate images of cells in a broad palette of colors, I am reminded of a friend's comment: "You know, a cancer cell is an object of beauty. It is elegant, a miracle of nature. It can do something other cells can't do. It can travel — an amazingly complex activity for a cell. Unfortunately, it is fine for the cell but destructive for the organism, because it has lost the capacity to live in harmony with its environment."

It is impossible to grasp the intricate complexity of the human body, a body created out of trillions of cells — a kaleidoscope of cells, multiplying in perfect sequence, all attuned to each other, all living in harmony. And then a renegade cell appears and boomerangs through the system, disturbing the order, the perfect balance. An invader, multiplying in rapid succession. Millions of microscopic genetic particles floating in a body gone haywire. A hidden disease that takes years to appear.

The imperfection of a perfect system — or is it the perfection of an imperfect system? Have these cells discovered the fault lines of the body's tissues, the weakened fissures? How does a mutant survive so long without detection?

Do the mystics believe that this too is in the nature of things?

On returning from a conference in New York, I was caught by the flamboyant colors of some photographs in an Air Canada magazine. David Doubilet, a deep-sea photojournalist, had written an article about a coral Eden off Bali. Describing the "submarine archipelagos" and the "tapestries of coral life," he writes, "I peer at the wrinkled exteriors of the largest sponges and, squinting, locate a pink fairy crab about the size of a penny, covered with white hairs. It skitters across its miniature moonscape, foraging on plankton that fall like dust on top of the sponge's rough surface."

I stare at the fairy-like decapod with its exquisite purple legs and coral-pink body. The Crab: Cancer in all her beauty.

"A woman can't feel cancer," says Zsigmond Sagi. "It starts in the body years before it is caught." In the folder labeled "Cancer," I find a title that catches my attention: "New Jersey Engineer Develops a Bra That Warns of Early Cancer by Measuring Body Heat." Alongside the heading, there is a picture of a man holding up a prototype of the heat-detecting pad and bra. Beside this picture is another one: the torso of a mannequin modeling the bra inserts.

The Hungarian-born engineer Zsigmond Sagi developed the Breast Cancer Screening Indicator (BCSI). According to him, the device, when tucked into a woman's bra, indicates an abnormality long before a lump can be felt. The non-reusable pads cost five dollars a pair. They are inserted into the cups of a close-fitting bra for fifteen minutes on the first day of the menstrual cycle. Sagi maintains that this is when a woman's body that has been going through hormonal changes returns to normal, and it is also an easy date to remember. Post-menopausal women can choose a random date each month, he says. Sagi's research was funded by Faberge, the cosmetics manufacturer.

Who is Zsigmond Sagi? Who could the inventor of such a device be? The article in *Publisher's Weekly*, from June 1980, describes him as a man of numerous inventions. He developed the zigzag Skip-Stitch for the Singer Company and opened Arden Laboratories (not to be confused with the cosmetic company) in Whippany, New Jersey, to develop and market tabletop soccer games.

When his father died of lung cancer in 1978, Sagi, an unrepentant chain-smoker, vowed to find a means of combating the disease. "He is confident his BCSI will revolutionize breast cancer detection methods," the article reads. It concludes with Sagi's words of advice for cancer patients: "I have eliminated the word 'impossible' from my vocabulary. Everything is possible. I have to believe what I'm doing. It's the only way."

After I read this article, I wondered if Zsigmond Sagi was still alive and what he was doing. My queries were answered when I sought out his name on the Internet. In the October 1997 issue of the *Journal of the National Cancer Institute*, there is an article on Sagi's research on the impact of temperature-sensitive pads in the detection of breast cancer.

• • •

It is my friend Gloria's birthday and I decide to arrange a birthday celebration. The summer heat suggests a Mediterranean menu: spanakopita with goat cheese and spinach, rice pilaf, Greek-style lemon potatoes, and Moroccan couscous salad with apricots and peanuts.

Gloria is radiant as she welcomes in her fiftieth year. We raise glasses of Chardonnay and clink a toast over the candles.

"To more birthdays."

"To the millennium, why not?"

"To life."

"L'chaim."

"Salut."

"Skol."

Gloria and Danny are talking about genetic disorders. Danny's research on genetic testing has earned him international fame. I hear his small hands tap the table as he absorbs the impact of Gloria's comments.

". . . and so my friend went for genetic testing as a preventive measure against breast cancer. And yet I understand that only ten percent of all breast cancers are genetic. So what's the point? Why don't they start spending more funds on the non-genetic factors, the other ninety percent?"

Legs in stirrups. Pelvic exam. In the Tao of sex, a woman's genitals are referred to as a "magic jade flower." I am exposing my magic jade flower to Dr. Ellen Buchman. She reaches inside me and I feel a twinge. Every year, it's the same routine.

"Okay, we're done," she says and I slide off the table.

"Anything new?" she asks, as I slip into my clothes and sit down beside her desk. Ellen is friendly, inviting in her approach. I have known her for five years. She does not insist on formal titles; I feel as if I am talking to a friend.

"Well, my sister has just been diagnosed with breast cancer, in situ. Early detection, positive prognosis. She had a lumpectomy and has just completed radiation therapy. Her oncologist has suggested genetic testing for her and her daughters. Her doctor mentioned that I might want to pursue this as well. Linda thinks I should definitely have it done."

"Well," Ellen says heavily, "you've certainly got the family history to suggest testing. But let's think this through."

I'm listening, breathing shallow.

"If you go for testing, will you be prepared for the results, and will you be prepared to act on them? If the results are negative, no problem, that's great. It doesn't completely rule out breast cancer for you, but you would deal with that situation if it arose. However, if the results are positive, then there is an eighty percent chance of a diagnosis of breast cancer and a fifty percent chance of a diagnosis of ovarian cancer. The recommended procedure is a prophylactic double mastectomy and a hysterectomy. The question is, will you be prepared to act on this finding?"

Words soar like black crows, hit the ceiling, and collapse at my feet.

"Think about it, Mavis. If you don't act on the findings, then you wait in suspense."

There is nothing to think about, a voice inside me thunders. "No, Ellen. There is nothing to think about," I blurt out.

"You don't have to decide today. We can discuss it again at a later date. In the meantime, here are some forms for the lab downstairs."

I stand, and feel like sitting down again. I regain my balance and leave the office, clutching the requisition for blood work.

I never pursued the genetic testing. My sister's cancer was, fortunately, detected very early. To date, she has had no recurrence. But I continue to worry about the genetics of cancer. The evidence is uncertain, inconclusive. In every group I facilitate, men and women become teary-eyed as they discuss their children — the sense of failure, the fear of transmission of a defective, mutant gene. Not only the burden of the disease, but the onus of a genetic legacy.

I hear their voices: "Why not my mother's beautiful auburn hair, my father's slim frame? Why not my natural affinity for sports, for music, for gymnastics? Why not her father's brains or intellectual curiosity? Why do I have to worry now about my flawed genetic markers?" Or, "I feel like a failure. I have brought my child into a world with the promise of care and safety. Now I may be abandoning them with an early death, and on top of that, I have to worry about my lousy, damaged genes."

My mother and I are sitting in the kitchen of her bright condominium with its blooming cacti, flowering cyclamen, and a vase of fresh-cut tulips and freesias. The sun is sparkling off the kettle. My sister has just had her surgery.

"I hope you are going to be tested. I hope you are going for regular checkups and breast examinations and I hope you are smart enough to have yearly mammograms." Her face is once again pale and drawn as she continues, "Linda's girls will have to be checked regularly, too. Maybe you can speak to them, Mavis. You know about these things from your work."

I nod in agreement, my face buried in the newspaper.

• • •

Crustacea is a subphylum of the animal phylum Arthropoda. Crabs, lobsters, shrimps, and wood lice are the best-known crustaceans, but the group also includes

> an enormous variety of other forms without popular names. Crustaceans are generally aquatic and differ from other arthropods. . . . Because there are many exceptions to the basic features [of Crustacea], a satisfactory inclusive definition of all the Crustacea is extraordinarily hard to frame. . . . Malacostracans (lobsters, shrimps, crabs, scuds, and pill bugs) . . . are the most numerous and most successful of the four major classes of Crustacea. Their members constitute more than two-thirds of all living crustacean species. . . . Malacostracans consume virtually every available kind of organic matter, plant or animal, living or dead.
>
> — ENCYCLOPEDIA BRITANNICA

In Dahab, a coastal oasis south of Eilat on the Gulf of Aqaba, I wait for Chaim. I sit in the shade of a palm grove, drinking my *caffe Americano*, as I watch a Bedouin in tight jeans and a kaffiyeh pick his teeth with the end of a match. He notices my gaze and smiles back at me, exposing a row of black teeth. I return to my reading about man's acquaintance with Crustacea.

W. Schmitt wrote,

> Early man — perhaps the Babylonians sometime about 2100 BC — translated the crab to the heavens, putting it in the zodiac as the sign of the constellation of Cancer. On every map of the northern hemisphere of sufficient scale the "Tropic of Cancer" is noted: Tropic, from the Greek word for the turn or change which marks the most north-

> ern limit on the earth's surface at which the sun may be directly overhead and at which the sun seems to pause before retracing its course to the south; and Cancer from the "crab" constellation. It is when entering this constellation that the sun is said to be at its summer solstice — the point in its apparent path at which the sun is farthest from the equator, in northern latitudes. The crab constellation is also called the "dark" constellation and is supposed to represent the powers of darkness.

Apparently the constellation was so named because the sun had a habit of traveling sideways like a crab while returning from its northernmost point.

Around me the calm sea relieves the ruggedness of the mountains. Chaim appears in silhouette through the haze of afternoon heat. I recognize his curly hair, his low-slung shorts.

"*Salaam, habibi,*" he greets me in Arabic style. We are Israeli travelers in a foreign land. "A great day to set out." He bends over and kisses me lightly on the cheek.

I am beginning a journey into southern Sinai. Chaim, a friend from my sojourn in Israel, has decided to meet me before I join my traveling group. An eclectic scientist, Chaim takes nothing for granted. He attempts to understand the complexity of life, making few assumptions. His work in genetics has deepened his respect for and humility about nature's mysteries.

"Why do you think the Crab was called the dark constellation?" I ask, still preoccupied with my reading.

"Perhaps because they burrow deep into the mud swamps

and watercourses of the river," he replies, without hesitation.

"But what about this guy?" I ask, brushing a sand crab off my toe. The crab scurries into the broad sweep of the landscape, hurtling its body across the sand.

"It is reluctant, that one. It wants to race to the sea. A bit lost, I would say." Chaim reminds me that crustaceans have a definite preference for marine environments, but that there is hardly a habitat type on the planet in which they cannot exist. "Amazing creatures. They can survive anywhere and can adapt to any habitat. There are also more species of these creatures than any other type — something like twenty thousand species."

Twenty thousand known species, multiplying in random succession across seven continents, in the depths of four oceans. I wonder if we shall be overrun by crabs one day.

• • •

Glenna, who has metastatic cancer of the colon, says that cancer cells thrive in acidic environments. "It is important to have an alkaline diet," she informs the group members.

The others resist. A diet with no herbs, no salt, no sugar, no oil — what does that leave? Steamed vegetables and boiled meat?

Sharon quietly speaks up. She is the nutrition specialist in the group. "How about chicken boiled in tomato cocktail on a bed of parsley and green onions? Or goat meat, that's permissible. Goat meat basted with cumin and lemons."

Glenna nods in agreement. She is attempting to create an internal ecosystem that is toxic to the cancer cells that inhabit her colon and stomach. She tells the group about ozone therapy, a form of treatment that is known to have positive results with certain forms of cancer. "Cancer cells hate oxygen. In ozone therapy, O_3 breaks down into O_2 plus an extra O, causing an excess of oxygen. This will choke out the cancer cells, or at least, that's the theory."

Chaim would listen intently when I talked about my work with cancer patients. He would try to understand the more human elements of my clinical work. Chaim was ten years older than I was. We met at a party when I first arrived in Israel for a ten-month sabbatical. Joking over cocktails, he called himself an evolutionary humanist. I said I was just a human revolutionary, and we laughed under the moonlight on a terrace in Ashdod. Then we walked down to the seashore and stared at the constellations etched against the black sky.

"An X-ray of the celestial body," I said, and Chaim bent over and kissed me lightly on the forehead.

"*Yiyeh tov, poh* [You'll be okay here]," he said in Hebrew, words that I learned only later. Words that captured the strained optimism of Israelis in a kind of national secret code.

Chaim's busy life in the south kept him occupied, but he managed to wrap a protective cloak around me, checking in with regular phone calls and an occasional visit to Rechovot, where I was staying. Over coffee and *sufganiot*, we would discuss the biological principles of life. Or rather, Chaim would talk and I would listen.

"Life is a trade-off. We all breathe — the so-called breath of life. The real miracle of life is not that we survive, but that we don't kill ourselves in the process of living. We breathe in oxygen approximately fifteen to twenty breaths a minute, yet oxygen is a toxic molecule when it is unpaired. In order to make use of oxygen, we must take in O_2, separate it, and recreate an active single atom with an active electron, while at the same time preventing it from causing damage. So being an oxygen-breathing organism is a delicate balance. In fact, an oxygen atom with an unpaired electron is asking for trouble."

It was Chaim who first explained the genetics of cancer to me. He told me that cancer cells are essentially normal cells that go wrong. They become an enemy from within, an autoimmune disease, unlike viruses or bacteria, which are external enemies that thrive on the host organism.

"Cancer cells attack healthy cells and become part of the new cells," he said. "They enter the genetic code and begin to multiply rapidly, like a machine gone out of control. Viruses, on the other hand, develop a symbiotic relationship with their host. Kill the host and you kill the virus. The treatment strategy for viruses is not to kill the healthy host cells, which is why viruses are often chronic. But in treating cancer, it's more effective to kill the healthy cells, because cancer cells share more features with healthy cells than virus-infected cells do."

One time, Chaim took me to Ein Gedi, a well-known nature reserve. As we hiked along the trail to the waterfall, I counted three ibexes, three hyraxes, and five goats. We picnicked at a small spring, Ein Shulamit, where there were no other tourists or hikers.

As we sat eating our pita sandwiches of cheese and cucumber, Chaim's face took on an intense expression. His jaw line dropped, narrowing his salt-and-pepper beard, and his bushy eyebrows formed a horizontal line across his forehead.

"You must know the second law of thermodynamics, a good Freudian like you. The second law states that energy will equilibrate somehow or the entity will become disordered. So life is about fighting entropy, fighting disorder. See this little crab here? He is fighting the fundamental law of the universe: to die. And so it is with every individual cell in our body. Every second of every day, some of our cells are receiving insults from the environment — from radiation, from DNA damage, from other agents. Eventually these cells are no longer able to replicate. Fortunately, our cells have an innate capacity to repair themselves, just like this guy here scurrying under the rock. But not all the damage can be fixed, and so some minor alterations may cause genotypic changes. These changes make the cell more vulnerable to further damage or intrusion.

"This is the so-called multiple-hit theory of cancer. These damaged genotypes become one hit in a cascade of events that causes cancer. It takes at least two hits, or changes, to the genes in the cell. These hits build up and interact over time until a breaking point is reached and cancerous growth is switched on. Get it?"

"Got it," I respond, clasping his large hands.

"Well, the hits may come from chemical or foreign substances that cause cancer, the so-called carcinogens that initiate the cancer process. These are the initiators. Or the hits may be promoters, which accelerate the growth of abnormal cells. What is critical is the number and type of hits, their frequency and their intensity."

"So what are the promoters and what are the initiators?" I ask.

"The initiators are substances like tobacco, X-rays, certain hormones and drugs, and excessive exposure to sunlight. The promoters include stress, which may weaken the immune system."

"But what about all the recent talk about environmental factors — diet, pollution, chemical toxins? The ecological corruption of the planet — how does that factor into the equation with all these promoters and initiators?"

"Not so simple. It's called genetic responsivity or genetic sensitivity. Our unique, individual responses to these so-called external agents are also genetically determined. It's the old nature/nurture mannequin dressed up in different clothes.

"So here we are in the middle of Ein Gedi and you are privileged enough to receive a private lesson in Cancer 101. And our little crab friend has probably disappeared from boredom or suffered cosmic damage from the sun's rays and gone home for a siesta."

"This reminds me of a comment made by a patient of mine. She said, 'Cancer hogs the conversation, manipulates the rules of social etiquette. I meet a man, a stranger in a bar, and as soon as I mention I have cancer, there is nothing else left to discuss. By the end of the evening, he knows all about me and I learn nothing about him.' And now cancer is hogging our afternoon hike."

I loved Chaim's flexibility, his ease in moving from one topic to another without a change in voice, pitch, or intonation — an adaptable, elastic mind. On our last visit together, we strode along the beach of Tel Aviv at sunset, collecting sand and seaweed between our toes. We walked all the way to the old port of Jaffa, talking about the Labour Party's decline in popularity and the growing number of settlements on the West Bank, about tattoos and body-piercing, Chava Alberstein's concert in Ramat Aviv, and all the other topics we regularly shared during our times together.

"One more theory," he said, as we settled into chairs at an outdoor restaurant. "This will be your last lesson. Then I will have taught you almost everything I know.

"Evolutionary biologists have a theory called 'the edge of chaos.' Organisms that are going to do well in life are those that live on the edge of chaos. What it means is that an organism must be as adaptable as possible — we call it living as far from the edge as possible — in order to be tolerant of environmental changes. Yet, at the same time, organisms must not be so modified or flexible that they are incapable of living day to day, carrying on the business of replicating, functioning, and so on.

"Multiple organisms like humans live at the frontier. We are forever being challenged to bend and adapt. Yet we are still not too far out on a limb to maintain our daily work. A fine balance, wouldn't you say? Living on the edge — not too far out, not too far in."

"And then again, there are some of us," I laughed, "who are way *over* the edge, even making it to the other side."

"End of lessons. You will probably be glad to no longer hear my lectures. But then again, you are such a receptive audience."

I knew I would miss Chaim, miss the warmth of his affection, his crooked smile and wild face, his sun-baked intensity and sense of humor . . . and most of all, his speeches.

• • •

The fossil record of the Malacostraca extends from the

> early Paleozoic era (Early Ordovician epoch, 505 to 478 million years ago) to the present. . . . The first eucaridan malacostracans appeared in the middle Paleozoic (Late Devonian epoch, 374 to 360 million years ago). These were burrowing, lobsterlike, protoglyphaeids with primitive, somewhat pincerlike walking legs and a tail fan. . . . During the late Paleozoic . . . malacostracans evolved rapidly. . . . At least 16 new orders [including the Decapoda] arose during that time. . . .
>
> Although malacostracans are typically free-living, several . . . among the . . . decapods . . . have formed symbiotic, commensal, and even fully parasitic relationships with other invertebrates. . . .
>
> — ENCYCLOPEDIA BRITANNICA

Nagar-Assura, workman of the riverbed. A clay tablet dating back to 500 BCE has been dug up in the valley of the Euphrates. Etched in cuneiform characters, the constellation of the fourth month, the Crab, is depicted under the name Nagar-Assura. A specialist in the field suggests that the common crab indigenous to the region's Mediterranean watersheds and islands, extending eastward into Mesopotamia and southward into Egypt and the Sahara, was likely the variety known as *potamon*. The Babylonians subsequently pushed potamon into the heavens.

The ancient Greeks had a different explanation for the constellation Cancer. According to Greek mythology, Hera sent a crab to nip Hercules between the toes as he was about to strike Hydra, the many-headed serpent. After Hercules crushed the crab under his foot, Hera raised it to a celestial place among the stars as a reward.

Potamon, the freshwater crab of the Mediterranean, is said to have traveled along the early routes of civilization. The human body has evolved its own routes: circulatory, lymphatic, pulmonary. Does cancer spread along the routes of least resistance? Or does it travel randomly through the body's canals?

One day, Nathalie said, as she clutched her abdomen, "I eliminate this route by surgery, and sure enough, it pops up somewhere else. It is determined to get me." Nathalie says that when she visualizes her attack on cancer, she imagines a floating seascape of traveling cells journeying to find new supplies of nutrients. In her visualization, she cuts off their food supply and dismantles their trade routes.

Breast cancer metastasizes from the breast to the lungs, liver, bones, or brain.

Pancreatic cancer metastasizes to the small intestine, bile duct, stomach, spleen, colon, and lymph nodes. Distant metastases may occur in the liver and lungs.

Squamous-cell skin cancer metastasizes to the bones, liver, and brain.

Uterine sarcomas can grow locally to involve the tissues surrounding the uterus and cervix, to the rectum and bladder and to the groin, pelvic, and aortic lymph nodes.

Colorectal cancer metastasizes through the lymphatic system to nearby lymph nodes, to the liver through the portal vein, and less frequently, through the bloodstream to the bones or lungs.

• • •

Ain Hudra, an oasis at the western end of the sandstone belt below the Tih plateau. It is March. In the early morning light, metallic flashes of copper and gold welcome the sun over the horizon. A group of urban nomads is being led into the south-eastern Sinai Peninsula by an Israeli guide and a tiny, ebony-skinned Bedouin named Ahmed. Time is suspended, measured only by the light and heat of the heaving desert.

I follow in Ahmed's miniature footprints. Walking beside me is a sabra with long legs and a Chicago Cubs baseball cap. His name is Nuri. He is a forty-four-year-old engineering foreman from Arad, once married and now separated. He recites these facts as if reading a script. He then goes on to tell me that the Negev is a more gracious desert than the Sinai, that his wife has just left him, that the Israeli guide is incompetent, that he is tired of lazy Arab workers, that he would like to visit America some day, that he is worried about the Israeli economy, that he is tired of reading about all those American peaceniks demonstrating in front of the Israeli consulate in Washington — after all, what do they know about the Palestinian question, and besides, if they are so concerned why don't they simply move to Israel and put their money where their mouth is . . . His words ramble on in an endless monotone, drowning out the stillness of the landscape.

I decide that he must be used to talking — to his wife, to his workers, to his children. I wonder if that is why his wife left him. I pretend to trip on a pebble and stop to clear my sandal, hoping that he will carry on without me. He keeps walking without interruption. I straighten up, regain my balance, and look ahead to see his head still bobbing and his arms still gesticulating.

Nuri is continuing his monologue with the young tourist from Australia.

I fall behind and Nuri's voice gradually dims. I listen to the grandeur of the desert speak in hushed pastel tones. I am surrounded by steep, high mountains. Rock formations of scarlet, pink, and purple are streaked with dark green, ebony, and red from the flows of magma that forced their way up through fissures in the rocks. Sharp, rugged peaks alternate with steep rock walls. A majestic display of shapes and colors. The towering slopes suggest fortifications against intruding marauders, a battlefield of giants hurling boulders at each other. How does life survive in these inhospitable surroundings of massive granite and schist? What master plan could there be in this landscape of both beauty and hostility?

Water supports the scant clumps of acacia and tamarisk and the palms of the oases — the very same water that is also a source of destruction. At times, torrential downpours rush unpredictably between the rock walls, sweeping away all that subsist: grasses, shrubs, trees, houses, animals, and people. A Chagall landscape of a world turned upside down. New growth and destruction. Life and death.

I look down at my feet. My boots are covered with the dust of the desert sands. Moonwalking. I wonder if there is life beyond this majestic scene in which the light displays a canvas that changes with movement — movement of my feet, of the sun and the moon, movement of the shifting of the universe as it tilts and sways beyond man's dictates. Across the bleached pebbles I notice a crab dancing sideways. Where does it live, this clever crustacean that can survive these conditions? Where is its home? Does it (he? she?) worry about survival or the meaning of life?

The group pushes on through the midmorning heat. As the sun shifts slowly overhead, Ahmed points to a canyon, an elephantine maw a hundred meters ahead of us. Without hearing his words, I know that we will stop beneath the coolness of the canyon ledge to rest. Time is not measured by clocks here in the desert, only by the intensity of light and heat.

In writing about Egypt, Susan Brind Morrow says, "If the city [Cairo] was Um A Dunya, Mother of the World, what was the desert? The city's negative: a blank page on which things magically appeared."

We stop for lunch, outstretched on the layered rocks. The landscape here is bare, devoid of plant life, without forests or lakes. The bedrock lies exposed, under constant attack by the elements. Green survives only where water accumulates after the flashfloods.

One of the Australian girls hands me a tin of hummus and some pita. I put my canteen between my feet and try to balance everything. Oranges taste sublime in the heat. I spread some hummus on my pita and lick my fingers.

Nuri has stopped talking. The others gather around the map to look at the rest of the day's route. Right now, we will eat. Then we will have our afternoon *hafsakah* perched on the shaded ledges, stretched out on the cool rock like animals. The warm water does not quench our thirst in the midday sun.

The light melts the colors of the canyon. I know that in a few hours the palette will change, for it is only at dusk and dawn that the true magic of the desert emerges in an arabesque of refracted light. Reds, oranges, pinks, and yellows — the poetry of the land.

The Sinai Peninsula, which forms a land bridge between Asia and Africa, was shaped by disturbances deep inside the earth's body. Sinai lies between two huge faults, branches of the rift valleys extending from Africa to Turkey. The Gulf of Aqaba is a deep scar on the earth's surface, produced by strong faults that led to the formation of the rift valley system. Enormous blocks of the earth's crust lie under the gulf. The steep scarps along its coasts indicate the main faults. The weakened rocks along the fault lines were easily eroded, which led to the formation of numerous wadis, or dry river beds, parallel to the coast. Further faults cross the eastern part of the Sinai Mountains, which also became fissured.

The earth's body, eroded and scarred by the massive forces of Mother Nature. An autoimmune reaction? A permanent mutation of the earth's landscape? Are fault lines responsible for the land's weaknesses and scars?

Continental drift was the creator of the Great Divide.

The world is divided into men and women. There were 15,119,439 men and 15,434,377 women in Canada as of July 1999.

The world is divided into those who have cancer and those who do not. It was estimated that in 1999, 129,300 people would be diagnosed with cancer in Canada. Of those, 66,500 would be men and 62,800 would be women.

The world is divided into those with prostate cancer, lung cancer, colorectal cancer, lymphoma, melanoma, leukemia, brain cancer, pancreatic cancer, multiple myeloma . . .

The world is divided into those who have a partner with cancer, a friend with cancer, a parent with cancer, a child with cancer, a colleague with cancer . . .

The world is divided . . .

5

In the anonymity of the consulting room, I listen to the words of my patients. I attempt to decode the cryptogram, the secret code of their inner worlds. Each patient speaks a unique language. For twenty years now, I have been sitting and listening to the outpouring of words that wash over me. What is the feeling that seeps into me? What are the colors of the words, the textures? Do the words threaten or intimidate? Do they seek solace or reassurance? Do they invite disdain or disaster? Are they welcoming or attacking?

Some words have a louder resonance, making themselves heard by their intensity and volume. Others are like a refrain, insinuating themselves through repetition: "I am egotistical"; "I am a freak"; "I am a lone ranger." But most of the words and phrases have a hidden history that is unknown to the listener, and that only becomes apparent through the shared dialogue of the therapeutic relationship.

Jacques Lacan wrote in a well-known statement that the unconscious is structured like language — a language with rules, structure, and precision. I imagine the unconscious as a text, and buried within the text, I visualize strands of beads, each forming a signifying chain that holds the essence of an undefined core. I imagine the unconscious as strings of DNA, like a genetic code.

I imagine the unconscious as a sunken treasure chest encased in mud, swallowed up by the bottom of the sea. I see some of its valuable contents, strands of diamonds, loosened and tossed about by the motion of the waves, the life force that expresses the sea's power. And every once in a while, I imagine the diamonds floating to the surface, dancing on the water in a display of brilliance — but alas, only momentarily, flashing briefly before sinking back into the depths from which they arose.

At night I play with these images in my mind. I think about the words of my patients. Each one of us has a style, an idiosyncratic speech pattern. We do not consciously think about this aspect of our speech, nor are we necessarily aware of it. And yet it exists, as clearly as our color preferences.

Thomas is a hairstylist who has an interest in body-work. He studies shiatsu massage and reiki, he has a black belt in tae kwon do, and he rides his bike to and from work daily throughout the year. In his sessions, he talks about the value of exercise, rest, and healthy eating. He eats organic foods, avoids caffeine, and swallows VegeSil, beta carotene, vitamin C, and devil's claw capsules twice a day. He frequently tells me that he loves his body, that he is proud of his physique, and that he is considering joining a nudist colony so that he can share in the pleasures of exposing his body with others. When he talks about himself, he refers to psychic scar tissue, memories stored in his DNA, arthritic relationships, and the need to eradicate the bacteria of his past. His language contains the images that are important to him.

One day, Thomas tries to convince me that he has resolved his relationship with his mother, with whom he has been fighting for several months. He offers up words on a platter of theories and explanations. He begins by describing his mother. "She is a Teflon woman. Everything bounces off her. Nothing lands and sticks. She is so sloppy."

I notice that he has moved away from the organic images of his regular speech. "Why sloppy?" I ask. "What does sloppy mean?"

"I feel shame somehow," he responds.

"Shame?" I repeat emphatically.

And he explodes, shaking his index finger at the air. "Shame on you, Mother, for being so sloppy, so out of control! Shame on you for walking to the door unclothed, unkempt, in front of me and my friends!"

A word. One word, *sloppy*. Words can open caverns within us.

I have learned that there are many different ways of listening. When I lived in Israel and was struggling to learn a new language, I realized that my attention was sharpest in the morning and weakest at night. During the day, my mind would try to decipher the elliptical vowels, the sharp consonants, parsing the run-on trail of words into small chunks. My whole being was engaged in a process of mental digestion, focused on the nuances of sound modulations. I would return home from a morning excursion to the supermarket, bank, or post office exhausted from concentration. But in the evening, as I sat in some café, cigarette smoke trailing into the steamy air and a singer stirring up rhythms in the corner of the dimly lit room, my mind would drift in and out of the Middle-Eastern melodies and minor chords of words whose meanings eluded me.

In my work as a psychotherapist, I am bombarded with information. Patients pour out the contents of their conscious minds. They tell me stories about their childhood families, their marital duos and trios, their relationships at work, intimacies of lives lived and living.

When I begin a session, I enter a domain of privacy. There is an intimate feeling about the world of listening into which I am transported. I sit in my comfortable wingback chair and let my eyes relax. I adjust my body until my shoulders drop and my feet are solidly planted on the footrest. And then I begin to listen.

When I listen to my patients, I try to unfocus, to not listen, to listen by disengaging from the immediate, the obvious. I look for the detail that is out of place. I listen for what does not belong. I wait for the obscure, the unnoticed — the slip of the tongue, the unwanted phrase, the discounted metaphor. The leg-tapping, the pause at the end of the sentence, the unabashed sigh.

As I sit, listening without listening, in a state of reverie, I hear the tragedies of daily life played out within the four walls of my room. I sometimes close my eyes to hear the gasps, the complaints, the tears — as well as the laughter and triumph of the human spirit.

When I listen to younger people, those aged eighteen to thirty, not only is my attention fully present, but I am also transported back to my own adolescence and young adulthood. I have a particular affinity and tenderness for the young people who come to the "I'm Too Young" group that meets at Wellspring weekly for eight to ten weeks. In one of those support groups, I met Julia and Sheila, Ashley and Marlene. At our first session, we talked about the meaning of life, and about death and the strangling web of cancer.

• • •

On the evening of the second I'm Too Young meeting, a young woman named Ashley appears twenty minutes early — a scrawny, bird-like apparition with red lips outlined in black, spiky hair tarred black, and the body of a concentration camp survivor. She introduces herself in a strong, deep voice and says that she is here for the young adult group and that she is sorry she missed the first meeting but she was out of town. She apologizes for her absence, hoping that it will not be a problem for the group.

I welcome her in to have some tea and show her which room we will be meeting in. I try not to stare as she walks in front of me, a narrow frame of stacked bones outlined by black tights and a black tank top. I figure that she has a stomach cancer that prevents her body from absorbing food. I know the others will also react to her appearance.

Later that evening, Ashley begins to tell her story to the

others. She does not cry. She does not flinch. She simply speaks the words, punctuated with her own rhythms, as though she were reading a book in which were recorded the details of a life lived, a life broken by misunderstanding and repaired by forgiveness.

"I was diagnosed with a brain tumor twelve months ago," she begins in her deep voice. "It's an astrocytoma. Funny word, eh? Well, the doctors couldn't figure out what I had for a long time, so when they finally found this thing in my brain, it was pretty advanced, eh? So I had radiation therapy five days a week for three months and I finished that six months ago. And my hair has grown back finally. Cool, eh?" She pauses and looks at the others as they all smile in agreement.

"So now I'm trying to get myself together. I've started painting and I've become very religious. I mean, not really *religious*, but spiritual, you know? So I see this minister regularly and we talk a lot. What about you guys?" She turns to the others again, as if all of a sudden self-conscious.

The others respond in turn. Julia, composed in her navy suit and tailored white blouse, describes her experience with a diagnosis of Hodgkin's lymphoma. She tells Ashley that she has returned to work — "That's why I'm dressed this way," she chuckles — and that she is hoping to get support from the group. She is upset about her father's death a year earlier. "Yeah, my father died from non-Hodgkin's lymphoma two weeks before I was diagnosed." She reaches for some tissues from the table.

Then Marlene quickly runs through her recent bout with the medical profession before they were finally able to determine that she has Hodgkin's lymphoma as well. "I'm just about to begin chemotherapy next week and I'm scared shitless. Same treatment as Julia."

And finally Sheila, who quietly and seriously says, "I also have a brain tumor, Ashley. It's a different kind than yours. It has a very long name, and because of my short-term memory problems, I can never remember it. I was attending McGill University in Montreal, but I had to move back here after I started having severe headaches and dizzy spells. One day I collapsed at school and was rushed to the hospital. My boyfriend had to call my parents. After my condition stabilized, I was transferred to Princess Margaret. But I'm much better now, only I can't go to school anymore. I still have some word problems and my eyesight is still poor. Occasional headaches and stuff."

Ashley rubs her forehead and then flicks her fingers through her hair as if to shake off some invisible flecks. When Sheila finishes, she speaks again. This time she talks more slowly and her words are bolder, pressing down like weights. "Five years ago, I began having pains in my feet. I complained and complained and the doctors insisted that they could not find anything wrong. Eventually I was sent to a psychiatrist, who said the pain was all in my head. I began having sessions with this shrink, who turned out to be a total jerk. He started giving me prescriptions and I started taking all these pills. They didn't make the pain in my feet go away and I began to get more upset.

"Eventually I ended up in the psychiatric ward of a hospital. I had to go to all these groups and I hated it. The only positive thing was the occupational therapy time, where I began to paint. And the weird thing is that I began to paint these shapes that resembled bodies, and in the head area were all these dark blotches. When I eventually saw the X-rays of my tumor many years later, it looked exactly like the blotches I had been painting. Maybe I'll bring them in some time.

"Well, as I said, I hated these groups and I especially hated this one therapist I had, who kept telling me that I had to eat more and that if I ate more I would not have the pain in my feet. She said I was anorexic. She said my problems had to do with my insisting on being estranged from my parents up north. Hey, they were my adoptive parents anyway, so why should I make the effort? They always said I was a big disappointment to them anyway. Besides, I've made contact with my real mom and I want to visit her.

"After several months, I got discharged from the ward. Nothing had really changed. I think they felt I was incurable or something. In any case, the pain never disappeared. I remember one day I could hardly walk because of it. But it wasn't until I threw up that I guess they began to do some other tests on me. That's when they found out I had this rare form of astrocytoma that begins with this foot thing. All this time, all those months of pain . . ." Her voice fades briefly.

"But after the radiation," she resumes, "I'm doing okay. I try not to focus on that. I think about the future now. I set little goals for myself."

It is hard to interrupt, to break this flow of optimism. I look around the room and Sheila's eyes are brimming. "You are amazing," she says, leaning over to touch Ashley's hand.

Marlene and Julia glance at each other. I do not know what they are thinking.

*

A week later. The weather has changed dramatically and a north wind blows the curled leaves into a heap by the front door. Walking creates new sounds, sounds that crunch, sounds that are not musical.

When I arrive, the Wellspring volunteer tells me that Marlene may be a few minutes late because she is tied up at work. Through the glass windows I see Sheila and Ashley engaged in conversation.

As I walk into the group room, Ashley asks me if it is safe to leave her bike parked in the alleyway. A pile of clothes lies in a heap beside her feet: fleece hat, gloves, vest, beige cable-knit sweater. "I'm back to my old means of transportation," she announces laughingly.

I assure her that her bike is safe and sit down to wait for the others. The fall chill unnerves me. This period of hibernation, of early winter retreat, haunts me with memories of my father.

The visualization exercise reduces the initial excitement and tension of the group's reunion. We go around the room reviewing the week, taking the group's pulse.

Julia begins, "It's the anniversary of my father's death this week. You know I mentioned that he had lymphoma, but he actually died of a brain aneurysm. It was awful . . ." Her voice stammers, stutters, as she reaches for a tissue. "I can't . . ." Again the pausing, the heaving.

I try to stay focused while Julia begins a third time. This time she is composed, like her tweed suit. "My family had to pull the plug. He was lying on his bed with tubes running in and out of his body. He no longer looked human. He was like a robot. I wanted to scream and pull him out of bed, to make him laugh, talk — anything to show me a sign of life. He loved life. He loved dancing to Fred Astaire in the kitchen, singing in the shower. He took us to the museum to see an exhibit on dinosaurs, because, he said, our history is embedded in the bones of the past. He loved all of it. And then to look at this man, this inert flesh, lying helpless on a hospital bed. My father . . ."

It takes Julia another few moments to compose herself. The group waits patiently, eyes downcast.

I looked out over the bobbing heads, my hand limp, people shaking my fingers, my hand disjointed from my wrist, my arm. I stood like a sentinel beside my mother, her face frozen in blankness.

I hadn't seen my father before he died. He simply fell down. Collapsed in a heap. Did he have a premonition? Did he know that this was to be his last dance, his farewell song? Did he reach for my mother or was she beyond his grasp? There are no details, only words: "Your father died." "He collapsed on the dance floor in a heap." I try to draw a picture, but I see only a heap on the floor.

The ambulance was called immediately, my mother reminded me. "There was a whole crowd of friends around him, just the way he would have wanted it. You know how social and outgoing your father was," she says. "Like he had a premonition and gathered everyone around to say goodbye."

"But I knew he was gone by the time the ambulance arrived," she continued. "I told the driver to go faster, but deep inside I knew he was gone."

Gone where? Where did she think he went? I never asked her.

I just held her hand in the cemetery. I held her hand while the snow made sparkling dewdrops on the fur coats, the yarmulkes, the stones, the earth, the mahogany box ("It's what your father would have wanted — mahogany"). I held her slim, cold fingers while the rabbi chanted an ancient prayer in an ancient language: *Yitborach, v'yishtabach, v'yitpoar, v'yitromam, v'yitnasay, v'yithador . . .*

My fingers were cold. I kept squeezing my mother's hand, hoping to spread life. But her fingers remained inert.

Week Four. Julia says she no longer knows who she is. She is confused and upset and trying to piece her life back together. Her treatments are over, her prognosis is good, but she has no energy. Her mother calls regularly, but she can no longer support her mother's emotional needs. "She pulls on me and I feel this weight on my shoulders. My massage therapist says I'm growing humps on my upper back and I —"

"Sorry I'm late," Marlene interrupts. "Tied up at work." She takes a seat beside Sheila. Julia's words hang in suspense.

"Well, I began chemo this week," Marlene continues. "Still have my hair, though. I was so panicky I could hardly sleep all week. My biggest problem right now is my mother. She's come zooming right back into my life, treating me like a five-year-old. She's so overprotective. I know she means well, but I'm twenty-eight, living with my fiancé and leading my own life."

"Mothers need to feel needed." Ashley speaks for the first time. "It's a maternal instinct or something like that."

"On the one hand there's my mother and on the other there's my best friend, who's avoiding me like the plague."

"I know that one, too. It's like people think cancer is contagious or something. You've got it and they think they can catch it or something."

"That's for sure."

For the next fifteen minutes, the group is engaged in back-and-forth conversation, bodies relaxed, sharing common ground. Then I notice that Sheila is quiet, distracted.

She begins, "My friends are scattered now. I was at McGill University in Montreal when my brain tumor was diagnosed in April. I began having severe headaches. The doctors thought it was migraines. Like you, Ashley, they kept sending me home, saying I was stressed from my exams. Then I collapsed in my apartment; luckily my roommate came in shortly after and called an ambulance. Apparently I had had a severe seizure. When I came to, my parents and boyfriend were standing around me as I lay in a hospital bed.

"I then had an operation that wasn't successful, because the tumor grew back, so I had another operation. I've just finished my radiation therapy and I'm beginning chemo tomorrow. I've had permanent damage to my peripheral vision and I have some residual problems with reading and writing, which should improve over time. I've been given five years by my doctors. I was initially devastated, but now I ignore it. I'm back here in the city and my boyfriend has transferred to the University of Toronto. We're living together now."

"Hey, is that the guy who dropped you off?" asks Ashley. "He's real cute."

"Yeah, that's him. He is so amazing. He wants to get married."

"That's wonderful," says Julia. "Roger is talking about marriage, too. Sometimes I wonder if it is a rescue thing, though. Maybe guys need to feel needed, just like mothers." And once again the atmosphere changes, bubbles of light breaking through the opacity.

Ashley looks tired today. She chats on about her friends and parents, casually mentioning that she was married and is now separated. "I dumped him. He was bad news — drugs and stuff. I no longer know what's normal. None of my life has been normal. I asked for my prognosis and I was given two to seven years. Well, I think those doctors just do guesswork. I don't even know why I asked. I kind of wanted to know, but now that I do know, I just ignore it."

Sheila says, "I do find that I want to do more things. At least, I wish I could if I weren't so tired. I'm volunteering at Mount Sinai Hospital on the neurological ward."

Julia sucks in her breath. "You are brave. That's gutsy of you."

During the rest of the session, Ashley and Sheila talk about their limited energy, while Marlene and Julia discuss what it's like to return to work.

During the week, I dream about my father. I am packing my suitcases for a trip I am about to take. As I look up to reach for a dress in the closet, my father appears, his body suffused with light. "Don't forget to take some warm clothes," he says. "It may get cold."

I am surprised by my father's comment, because I am leaving for a Caribbean island. I say, "Sure, Dad." But when I look up, he is gone.

I remember that Mrs. D., an East Indian patient of mine,

often dreamed of her dead brother in Bombay. She told me that, in her culture, when you dream about someone you love, it means that they need something from you. She said that she was psychic and that she had dreamed twice about her brother appearing to her.

I worry about what my father might be trying to tell me.

Week Five. Marlene's hair is thinning. Ashley is wearing a black miniskirt with black tights; an embroidered camisole shows under her sweater. Julia is leaning forward in her chair, while Sheila reclines with her long legs tucked under.

Sheila begins, "I began chemo this week. It's an oral medication. I'm even more tired now than before. I hate it. I hate that my boyfriend is busy at university all day while I have a hard time focusing on reading simple things. The words blur on the page and the letters get mixed up in my head. Since I've moved back to Toronto with him, I'm even lonelier during the day. I hate that I'm jealous of my friends who are still in Montreal having fun and partying. This is no fun, no goddamn fun." Instinctively Sheila covers her mouth, but the words have fallen out, tossed into the room like pulled-up weeds.

"We're all in the same position," Ashley says. "We're all too young. But we have to make the best of it. Right?"

"But it seems so unfair at times," Marlene joins in. "I alternate between being angry and frustrated and thinking that everyone is thrown something to deal with, so this is my package. I don't ask 'Why me?' anymore. I try to get on with it in some way."

*

Six months after my mother's first diagnosis of breast cancer, she sat down with me in the kitchen. Sipping her coffee, cup shaking slightly in her hand, she stared down at her plate and said quietly, "There's something I've been meaning to tell you."

I could feel my pulse quicken, my palms begin to sweat.

"I always thought about it, you know," she continued. "The cancer, I mean. I always thought I would get cancer like my mother, like Bubbe. Sometimes I even wonder if I made it happen — created it by worrying and thinking so much about it."

I could feel her gaze on my face as I toyed with my pasta salad. *Tricolor fusilli,* I thought. *It matches the sun-dried tomatoes and pesto sauce.*

"Do you think your mother is weird?" The words hung in the air. "My advice to you, my dear," she continued, "is not to think about it. Don't think about me and Bubbe. Protect your body. You mustn't ever think about it."

My mother's curse: an incantation, "Don't think about the cancer." Okay, I won't think about the cancer when I go for my annual checkup and the doctor pokes and kneads my breasts. I won't think about it when I book my annual mammogram and spend a morning in the Women's College Hospital Breast Imaging Department. I won't think about it when I prepare my lecture "Mothers and Daughters: Breast Cancer Prevention." I won't think about it when one more friend tells me about a friend, colleague, mother, or aunt who has just been diagnosed. I won't think about it when my sister tells me her physician suggests we go for genetic counseling. I won't think about it when my sister is diagnosed with breast cancer just before her fiftieth birthday.

*

Week Six. Julia says that she has had a better week. She went to the cemetery on Friday, stood beside her father's gravestone for a long time, and talked. She thanked the group for being so supportive. "I realized after that session several weeks ago that it was the first time I'd really talked about my dad's death. I felt awkward because I know we're here to discuss our own cancer. But somehow the two are so linked in my mind that I just had to talk about my father first."

Marlene speaks, dragging out her words. "This wasn't the greatest week for me. I'm beginning to feel some side effects from the chemo. It's mainly fatigue. Every Sunday night I get anxious thinking about Monday morning. My fiancé is so supportive that I sometimes feel guilty for putting him through this. We had to put our wedding off for a year. The invitations had already been printed. And the date was yesterday."

"Well, think about how much more meaningful it will be a year from now," Julia chirps up.

I sense that Ashley is restless, anxious to speak. "I've had a great week," she begins, her voice hurried. "I got a photo album with family pictures from my biological mother in Calgary. I'm hoping we will meet soon."

As usual, Ashley had surprised the others with this casual reference to her chaotic life. "My adoptive parents wrote me off a few years ago when I was diagnosed as being manic-depressive and anorexic at the same time," she continues. Sensitive to the raised eyebrows, she smoothly moves the topic sideways like a master chess player. She says she is planning to send her natural mother pictures of her in different wigs.

"You know, when I was undergoing chemotherapy, I would

visit my doctor every week in a different colored wig — black, blonde, purple. I loved to see his expression. And then I would have great fun with my clothes. Miss Flamboyant, they called me."

"That is so cool, Ashley. I wish I could be more like you. I guess I'm too inhibited," Julia says.

"No, you can do it, too. You have to let go. It's so much fun!"

"I'm not so sure my boss would like it if I showed up with five earrings, black nails, and Doc Martens."

"I guess I'm lucky that way. I don't have to worry about it. No job, no dress code."

It feels like a pajama party — fashion, cosmetics, jewelry, accessories. The group ends on a high note.

Week Seven. Today Ashley looks buoyant, her face still flushed from her bike ride to Wellspring. After the relaxation ritual, she leads off the group. "I brought something tonight, but I'm not sure I have the guts to show you," she begins.

"You must, you must," the others squeal like schoolchildren. "You brought it, so you have to show us."

"It's her artwork, I know it. She said she'd bring it one day."

"You absolutely *must* show it to us. We won't let you go otherwise."

Ashley reaches for her portfolio. She carefully lays it on the coffee table and slides out a stack of 30 x 36 inch sheets of paper. The group waits patiently. One by one, Ashley holds the pictures up in front of her.

Black background with green moon shapes. Circles of yellow light filled with intricate patterns of lines, like worms. Thick oils in deep ocher overlaid with dark green blotches. Filaments, amoeba-like tentacles, flowing beads, amorphous shapes.

The group is speechless. When Julia, Marlene, and Sheila regain their composure, they speak in hurried excitement.

"You have to do something with this stuff. It's fabulous."

"And you say you've never taken an art class? That's amazing. You're a natural."

"You absolutely must continue this work. It is so, so . . . *awesome*."

I join the group in their support of Ashley's work. As the group leaves that night, I hear Julia saying that she is going to sign up for an art class. I wonder whether she will have the energy to pursue her desire.

Ashley, Marlene, Julia, and Sheila hug each other as they leave. When I turn off the lights and step out into the parking lot, I can still hear their chatter and giggles — the sounds of life.

Week Eight. Sheila informs the group that she has had another seizure. In a frozen voice, she says that she has had to move back home again, that her boyfriend is being understanding, that her freedom is limited, that she cries when no one is around to hear her, and that she is fatigued and depressed.

"It was all going so well, and now this. Back to more medication, more tests, more monitoring, more nuisance. Fears and tears, I call it. I can't face my parents. I can't look into their faces. My mother ages visibly every day that goes by."

Ashley places her hand gently on Sheila's shoulder.

What is a seizure? A violent disease of the nervous system. A massive excess of involuntary action or emotion, marked by irregular contractions or spasms of the muscles, terminating with relaxation.

When I was in Grade One at Hampstead Public School, Roger Carmichael fainted during morning exercises. At exactly 9:10 a.m., as we sang the national anthem, Roger collapsed. After three such episodes, Roger was absent from school for a week. When he returned, he looked the same, but he no longer had to stand for the Lord's Prayer or "O Canada." Mrs. Laing told us (in front of Roger) that he had epilepsy, and we were given a brief lecture on what might happen if Roger had a seizure in class. In the playground at recess, Shelley Morris said she had seen her cousin have a seizure, and it was the scariest thing she had seen in her life. Roger continued to play soccer at recess, but he had to go home at lunchtime for the balance of the year.

The group is silenced by Sheila's news. Finally, Ashley says that she had a good consultation with her oncologist, but she is concerned about a freckle on her left shoulder. "I'm probably just being paranoid, but I can't help wondering if the cancer will return in some other disguise."

She then adds that she is anticipating a visit from her adoptive parents, who live near Timmins. They will be spending the weekend with her, and Ashley does not always relate well to them. "You know, I've put them through so much, and now this. They just don't know how to handle me, or it, or whatever. I used to be a real party girl — drinking, drugs, the whole bit. Then I also had a lot of problems in adolescence — panic attacks, agoraphobia, eating disorder. I was a mess. Now I just pray. I sometimes wonder if I'm being punished in some way for my past. So now I have these strong religious and spiritual beliefs. My minister visits me twice a week and we even pray together at times. I've stopped worrying about what others think. Masks — it was all masks." She stops suddenly, then laughs. "Listen to me, hogging the whole session."

Julia joins in her laughter. "You always amaze me, you really do."

Near the end of the session, the group returns its attention to Sheila. They offer her words of support. They know her situation is serious.

"This seizure has forced me to accept the reality of my cancer and my diagnosis. I know I will never be the same again, my old self. At times I have this sense of moral superiority, like I understand all about life and death and stuff. But then I think I'm kidding myself. If I were healthy, I'd be out partying and laughing with my friends, too."

Week Nine. My week has been difficult: another Wellspring death. A member of my current metastatic group has died and I have just returned from a viewing at the funeral home. There is a light dusting of snow on the ground. Winter hovers nearby. I am a few minutes late for the group.

When I arrive, I hear Julia and Marlene laughing in the kitchen area. Through the window I see Sheila sitting on the sofa, clutching a pillow to her chest. Ashley emerges from the washroom. "Hi," she says, her lips outlined in deep mahogany this evening. She hikes up her tights and follows me into the group room.

The session begins the way it does on any other night: visualization, check-in, back-and-forth discussion.

Julia: "Well, I got a clean bill of health. It was my six-month checkup and I'm doing okay. And it was my birthday yesterday, and my co-workers decorated my cubbyhole with balloons and bought me a cake."

Ashley: "I had a good week, too. I had good test results and I'm off my anti-seizure medication. Plus, my parents came and we had a good visit — conflict-free except for the usual nagging."

Sheila: "I had good news and bad news. The good news is that there is no change in my tumor growth. The bad news is that I'm going to have these problems permanently — the memory loss, the reading difficulties, the word-recall problems. It means that returning to university is out. My parents and oncologist are arranging for me to see some specialist in Ottawa."

Marlene: "I had a visit with my sister that was good. The chemo is going all right, but I still get very anxious and nauseous the night before my appointments."

The group continues to discuss changes in lifestyle, changes in relationships. They are respectful of each other; there is a positive tone.

And then Marlene says, "You know, I worry about the long-term impact of treatment. There's the risk of recurrence in ten to fifteen years, risk of heart disease, and the whole issue of children. Bill and I want to have kids after we're married. I was told we'd have to wait a few years before we try, because of the chemotherapy. Then, they say, it's safe. But I don't know if it's possible or not after chemo."

Julia adds, "I also worry about heart disease. I know I got a clean bill of health, but how do you ever forget the cancer when there will be these reminders in the future? We want to have kids, too. But we're not sure we can anymore."

As I look over at the others, I see Sheila and Ashley huddled into the sofa. Their eyes are glistening. Sheila begins to speak, her voice wavering, "Well, at least you can contemplate having children. You can think about ten to fifteen years from now. I've been given less than two years, and right now I believe it will be less than that. I have no future."

For the first time in two months, Ashley breaks down in tears, her black eyes smeared with black makeup. "And what kind of future do I have? I've been given two to three years to live. Children? How can I even dream of a future, let alone children? I . . ." Then her mouth snaps shut, like an oyster protecting its pearl. "I have my spiritual beliefs and they keep me going. I am glad for what I have."

Three pairs of eyes turn toward me. I invite Ashley to speak some more, to let it out, to rant, to cry, to open up again. But she has locked herself up, receded back into her shell.

The meeting ends in some discomfort. Ashley asks to speak to me. As we round the corner into the tiny Wicker Room (so named for its furniture), she says abruptly, "Mavis, I can't do this anymore. I'm not coming back."

"What do you mean?" I ask.

"I just can't do it. I hate crying. I need to be strong. I've said too much tonight and offended the others. I've done the group thing in the past, and it doesn't work for me. I can't allow myself to get depressed. I've worked too hard to get to this point. I have my beliefs . . ." Her voice trails off.

"I know the group wants you to stay. The week you were late, they told me how much you give to them and how much they admire you."

My words are too weak. They fall to the ground without making an impact. Ashley has already left the group. We say goodbye and I hug her skinny frame. I can feel her resistance to my embrace, her ribs protruding into mine.

"Ashley, if you change your mind, you know that you are welcome to come back any time," I call out the front door into the snow showers.

I try to call Ashley during the week, but I just get her voice mail. I try again before the last group session, to invite her to the closing party, but there is still no response. She once told me that when she is depressed she will not answer the phone. I imagine her lying on her bed, surrounded by oriental pillows and burning incense.

I try to piece together the fragments of her young life: adopted at a few months old by a pair of teachers living in rural northern Ontario; growing up as an only child with few friends; a turbulent and chaotic adolescence enveloped in a drug-filled haze; a series of psychiatric evaluations, hospitalizations, and treatments; making contact with her biological mother after being diagnosed a year before. When Ashley received the photo album from her natural mother, she was so excited, convinced they would soon be reunited.

"What is a normal life?" she once retorted when Marlene complained about the disruption that cancer and its treatment were causing. In Ashley's short life, she has mentioned ten years of mental suffering — manic depression, agoraphobia, panic attacks, anorexia, substance abuse. There were allusions to wild partying, a brief marriage, and lately, renewed contact with her ex-husband, who was now in a drug rehabilitation program. Everywhere lie scattered scraps of information, fragments of her life that she tossed out to the others. Only in the months just before joining the group has she found renewed faith in religion. She talked about a strong spiritual belief, a return to God's fold. A priest visited her regularly in her apartment, in addition to her weekly church attendance.

I am concerned about Ashley. I want her back in the group. There is both a vulnerability and a strength about her that I find endearing and engaging. She elicits a maternal, protective response in me. She has unwittingly seduced me into her life of heartache and pain. I recognize the signs of my rescue fantasy; there is always someone who plucks a bit harder on one's emotional harp.

The following week, the group discusses Ashley's departure. Sheila says that the word "future" has a different meaning for everyone. Julia and Marlene are mired in guilt about raising the issue of children. They continue to worry about their futures. The farewell party unleashes tears and laughter. The group promises to stay in touch.

Three months later, I learn that Sheila has died. I attend the funeral, signing the guest book with splotches of ink like floating clouds around my name. The chapel is full, congested. I find it difficult to breathe. I introduce myself to Sheila's parents and they stare at me with vacant eyes. "Yes, we have heard about you and the group. So helpful. Sheila talked about it," her father says.

I try to call Ashley once again. There is no response or voice-mail message. I do not know if she is still alive.

• • •

I am always struck by the resilience and adaptability of young people, their ability to forgive and move on, the energy and spirit that make working with young men and women such a rewarding experience.

For young cancer patients, there are recurrent themes of feeling cheated, of being too young, of the doctors' condescension to people their age. On the one hand, some physicians go out on a limb to make more of an effort for the future citizens of our society than for the elderly. On the other hand there are the groan-inducing, patronizing comments: "You're so young, you poor thing."

These young people, poised on the brink of their adult lives, have been thrown a monkey wrench. They speak honestly and openly about the strength they have gained from their diagnosis. They discuss the injustice of their destiny, their fears about dating, their renewed dependence on family at a time when they are supposed to be leaving the nest.

Last night a group was discussing views on spirituality. One member spoke about everything in life happening for a reason. This position was supported by another group member, who stated that she had become more spiritual since her diagnosis. She believed that her increased faith was a positive outcome of her diagnosis. Two other members shook their heads in disagreement.

"I wish I could believe that were the case. It would be a whole lot more comforting. I've had cancer once, and if there was a lesson to be learned, I'm sure I would have learned it then. So what about the second time around? What could possibly be the reason for a recurrence two months after my treatment ended? Was I that poor a learner? Did I miss something? As a result, I have no belief in god, no faith, no religion. I believe that a person dies and is buried. Period. End of story."

And yet, when this young woman described all the healing circles in the city that were praying for her, she said, "Well, of course that's okay with me. You never know what can happen." The uncertainty, the struggle for absolutes and truths — yet acceptance of compromise, of partial truths. The flexibility of contradictory positions.

It is hard not to feel touched by these young people. They elicit such powerful parental and protective responses. When I hear myself thinking, *They are too young*, I remember Sheila, twenty-one years old, saying, "I'm not too young. I've had a life. What about all those little kids at the Hospital for Sick Children who have cancer?"

• • •

Tupper, Fran, and I plan a reunion for the I'm Too Young program. Five years, ten groups, sixty people. Young people are nomads, wanderers, trying out new jobs, new perfumes, new domiciles. Locating sixty young adults in a large city, where change is as much a part of life as dressing, is no mean feat. Who could know how many had moved, how many had died? Did

Sarah make it after her surgery? Did Shelley survive her second round of chemo?

I harness my determination and begin calling. The phone calls are either curt or friendly, strained or engaging.

"Hi, Michael. It's Mavis . . ." Silence. "From Wellspring." Pause. More silence. Then recognition.

"Mavis . . . Wellspring . . . Wow, how great to hear from you!"

Or, "George?"

"Who is this speaking? George died six months ago. This is his father."

Twenty-five people respond to the invitation.

It is 6:45 p.m. and the reunion is to begin in fifteen minutes. Tupper and I are arranging trays of sandwiches and fruit platters that have been donated by a restaurant nearby. I have known Tupper for many years, watching him in the roles of member of one of the young adult groups, participant in the training program for volunteers, and peer-support volunteer. As with all the young adults, I admire his courage and determination, his vitality and energy in the face of his diagnosis. Today he has been in remission from Hodgkin's lymphoma for ten years.

After Tupper, Lisa is the first to arrive. Bracelets from her wrist halfway to her elbow, glistening lips, loosely tossed curls, and cowboy boots. We hug and I marvel at her physical strength. Lisa works in the film industry, marketing new talent. She speaks easily of films she has vetted, the upcoming film festival, the late-night parties of movie people. She is silent about her disease.

As I pour myself a drink, I feel a hand on my back. "Hi, how *are* you?" a voice blurts out. I turn to face Fran and we embrace, swaying silently in each other's arms. I have known Fran through two support groups. In the first group, she spoke few words, her eyes glazed, spikes of hair poking out of a red bandana. When she did speak, the words appeared to stick in her throat, forced out without emotion or punctuation. Dead words: "My name is Fran I was diagnosed with cancer Hodgkin's lymphoma Stage IV. I am undergoing chemotherapy six months it's been three months so far. I quit theatre school I have no life now just chemo just nausea just sleep and chemo."

A year later, Fran signed up for a second group. Her chemo had been successfully completed and she had returned to theatre school. It was Fran who taught me that endurance and dedication are worth the battle, that hard work produces results, that remaining faithful to your dream is what matters. Fran had a vision of being an actress. She nourished her talent by writing and earned money by carrying platters of food at a bistro on Yonge Street and answering the phone at an uptown fitness club. After much hard work and a concerted effort, Fran wrote, produced, directed, and acted in a play about her experience with cancer.

Fran is twenty years younger than I am. Her mother died from a heart-and-lung condition when Fran was fifteen years old. Her father lives out of the city. At times I want to wrap myself protectively around her, filling in where the maternal function was prematurely interrupted. Whenever we walk arm in arm down College Street or St. Clair or Queen Street West, investigating new cappuccino haunts and bakeries, I feel that life has unlimited possibilities.

I notice Tim squeeze between two chairs as he makes his way to the beverage table. Tim's shirt is crisp and his pants well pressed, with straight creases. His cane is folded up like a collapsible umbrella. As he approaches, he reaches forward to hug me and kiss me on the cheek. Paco Rabane . . . Tim loves to experiment with new fragrances.

Tim's brain tumor left him visually impaired. Against medical odds, he outlived his prognosis and began a new career, working with visually handicapped patients and volunteering at Wellspring.

The room fills up quickly, within twenty minutes it is buzzing with steady conversation. Party sandwiches, cheese, and fruit slices gradually disappear.

Shelley waddles over, her belly a container for new life. We hug and I feel the fullness of her pregnancy press against my middle. "It's for real," she says. "Seven months. We know it's a baby girl. Yes, there is life after cancer."

I do not need to hide my tears. "Congratulations. That's wonderful." And I hug her again.

Fran, Tupper, and I call the group to order. Tupper flicks the lights; Fran crosses her legs decorously and takes a sip from her Coke. I catch her eye and we smile. Everyone takes a seat, on the familiar sofas with the bold chenille prints or the burgundy chairs or the floral wingbacks.

When the sounds die down, I begin. "There are many things we have in common and many more that we do not. But I know we have all shared in the opening ritual of visualization, with my voice telling you it is okay to take a pause, to relax and let go. And so I want you now to allow your bodies to settle in your chairs, and when you are ready, invite your eyelids to close gently, easily . . ."

I hear the breathing — the breath of life, a chorus of sound.

It is written in Genesis 2:7 that "the Lord God formed man of the dust of the ground, and breathed into his nostrils the breath [*neshamah*] of life; and man became a living soul [*nefesh*]." According to the Alkalay Hebrew dictionary, *neshamah* is a vital need, the source of life. Breath is a connection to God.

It is known that the earth resonates at 7.8 hertz, which is equivalent to man's brainwaves in a state of calm breathing. It is also known that this electromagnetic pulse of the earth is equal to the human body's natural electrical field when it is in a healthy state of balance.

When I finish the exercise, I notice Mr. Cohen and Mrs. Tirkopolous standing by the doorway. I welcome them into the group. Mr. Cohen greets me with a smile; I notice that his peach-colored shirt is stained a deep tangerine at the armpits. Mrs. Tirkopolous, hair pulled back tightly in a bun, is dressed in black. She nods an acknowledgment in my direction.

Fran officially welcomes everyone. I am beginning to wonder about the impact of the setting on everyone when Wes blurts out, "Just like old times, only a bigger group."

"Yeah, it feels weird."

"But comfortable."

"Takes away the mystique. I was scared to come back here — too many bad memories. But it's cool."

"I'm relieved that I can walk in here and not be freaked out, too. I was kind of dreading the return back."

"Well, it's great to see all of you," I say, finding words too glib or mundane to communicate my excitement. "I just want to embrace each and every one of you." People smile and I am momentarily tongue-tied.

"Before we have a chance to share what has been happening, as part of this evening we would like to take a few moments to remember those who have died within the past few years," I say, removing a bag of colored candles from under my chair and placing it on my lap.

A glass bowl sits alone on the coffee table. It is filled with water, filled to the level of the grapes etched around it. Fruits of the vine. Offerings.

"First of all, a candle in memory of Paul Johnson," I hear myself say. "Who is from Paul's group? Who would like to light a candle for him?"

Lisa's bracelets jingle as she shakes her hand in the air. "I would," she says. "I was at his funeral and spoke there at his wife's request."

I know that Lisa and Carole, Paul's wife, were friends. I also know that Carole would have been here tonight if she hadn't moved to Australia with her six-year-old daughter. Lisa comes forward, lights a green candle, and places it gently in the bowl of water.

"Would anyone like to share some memories of Paul?" I ask.

"When I think of Paul," Laura volunteers, "I think of his discussion of statistics. 'I'm not gonna be a statistic,' he said. 'I want to go rock-climbing and parachuting and I want to have another child.' He was so full of life."

As I picture Paul in the group sessions, I hear his quiet voice struggling with the ethical decision about having a child. "I may not be here to help parent another child. Is it fair to the child, to my wife? And yet I feel this strong urge to have one more child. Do you think it is selfish to want to leave a legacy, a memento of my life?"

Others speak up, one by one, until the room returns to silence.

"And now a candle for Dahlia Cohen," I say. "Mr. Cohen, would you like to light a candle for your daughter?"

"Actually," Mr. Cohen replies, "I would be honored if Tim would light a candle for her."

I feel my eyes brimming as Tim walks over without his cane. "How about a pink one?" I whisper, as he fumbles for a candle. I help Tim light the candle and he places it gently in the bowl.

When Tim returns to his seat, he begins to speak. "Dahlia and I had the same diagnosis, so we developed a special closeness, relying on each other. I was a few years ahead of her in terms of diagnosis, but she would say, 'Dammit, if you can do it, then I can beat this thing, too.'"

"I remember how amazing she was. She continued going to York University to complete her year while she was undergoing treatment."

"And I remember how she began giving talks on cancer as a fundraiser so that she could feel she was helping others."

"I remember the time she . . ."

"And what about . . ."

Words of praise. Words of support. Mr. Cohen wrings a soggy tissue in his hands. His cheeks are moist and he wipes his eyes.

Slowly, with dignity, we move through the list of names, lighting candles and remembering: Paul Johnson, Dahlia Cohen, Sheila Horvath-Thurolzyne, George Gaynor, Sheila Stephenson, Bill Tirkopolous. The glass bowl of floating candles sparkles.

"And now it is time for the group to have an opportunity to share what has been happening in your lives," I say, after a respectful pause. There follow stories of success, of remission; stories of recurrence and further treatment; stories of births, of work promotions; stories of transformation and stories of living.

I stare at the glass bowl. Floating colors of death.

And what are the colors of life? I wonder. Rainbows, apple blossoms in spring, Niagara peaches in August, fields of lavender in Provence, red poppies sprouting from the clay sands of the Judean desert, sage-green lichen under the low light of the Arctic sun.

6

Daughters invisibly enter the room and slip into the chairs occupied by four adult women. The cast of characters:

Tove — a forty-eight-year-old woman with metastatic pancreatic cancer, dressed in baggy clothes that hide her skeletal body.

Lily — a fifty-five-year-old woman with metastatic breast cancer, dressed in a fashionable navy pantsuit with a floral scarf.

Carole — a fifty-one-year-old woman with metastatic breast cancer, dressed in comfortable loose pants, a sweater, and walking shoes.

Preeya — a sixty-three-year-old woman with metastatic

ovarian cancer, dressed in a tunic and trousers with a woolen shawl around her shoulders.

Mavis — the facilitator, dressed in black pants and a black sweater.

The scene — the fourth session of a twelve-week support group at Wellspring for people with metastatic disease.

The mood — unknown.

Carole begins by describing a childhood of merriment and affectionate hugs — making lace angels from spider webs; beading colored popcorn strands for the Christmas tree; dried roses and irises pressed between the pages of leather-bound classics: *Oliver Twist, Wuthering Heights, A Tale of Two Cities*; family vacations to Disneyland. "My mom and I would gang up against my brothers and my dad. There was a gender split, all right, the girls versus the boys."

Carole's voice drops and she crosses her arms over her chest. "But then, when I hit adolescence . . ." She pauses and sighs. "It all stopped. Suddenly, just like that," snapping her fingers. "It was as if I had become unsightly or unappealing or something. My mother wanted no part of me. The tickling, the laughter, the burnt marshmallows over the backyard campfire — it all stopped. It was like as soon as I became a 'woman,' she rejected me. I had become a monster with breasts. Or at least that's what my therapist suggested.

"It was the same way she handled my first period. She threw a box of Kotex into the bathroom and said, 'Here. Welcome to womanhood.' You know, I sometimes wonder if my mother's rejection of breasts is related to my breast cancer. In fact, in my mind there is a definite connection."

Carole falls silent. The group is considerate, pacing their comments.

Lily speaks next. "You know, Carole, I share a similar sentiment. I grew up in Guyana, a West Indian culture where women have no say. Even though my parents separated when I was older, I grew up silenced by my father's eyes, my father's brown leather belt, and the sound of my father's shoes on the entrance tiles. My mother was like a trapped moth, fluttering in the daylight hours and gathering strength in the evening when my father drank himself into oblivion.

"I lost a sibling — a blue-eyed baby brother — before I was born, and I became the 'replacement child,' the rescuer for my mother, the confidante, the garbage can. My father cursed the death of his son, heaping blame on my mother and her 'wicked voodoo body.' Sometimes I dreamed of being a boy. I thought a boy would arouse my father's love and desire. But instead, his wrath beat my mother into the ground, so far deep that I think she never saw the sun from where she was lying.

"I too have breast cancer. And I too wonder if my breasts are a part of my anatomy too rejected, too unwanted, too . . . to be cherished."

My hands perspire. I look at the others. They are rapt from the power of Lily's words. The two who have not yet spoken look at each other. They decide between themselves who will go next.

"Families —" Preeya begins. She coughs, clears her throat, slowly reaches for her water bottle, and sips until she is ready to speak.

"I grew up in Calcutta. Crowded city, yes? We were relatively well off. I was the second child of nine, the first girl. My father died when I was fifteen years old and my mother had all these children to feed. She pounced on me to help out. So I helped out with all the chores: pounding blankets, sweeping floors, cooking chapatis and mung dal, rice and aloo gobi. I vowed I would never have children, because I spent my teenage years babysitting and parenting. No, no children for me.

"Now I have one daughter — one daughter who is bulimic. In and out of psychiatric hospitals, living at home and watching her mother's belly swell with cancer. Ovarian cancer. You ask, 'Is there a connection?' I ask the same question."

It is Tove's turn to speak. "Well, I might as well tell you the whole story. I grew up in Denmark. Copenhagen — wonderful, wonderful Copenhagen," and she repeats the phrase in Danish, lengthening the vowels.

"My mother and father separated when I was very young, two years old. My sister, who was four years older than me, went to live with my father. There was no contact with him after the first six months of their separation or, for that matter, with my sister. I grew up thinking I was an only child. My mother never said a word about my having a sister living in the same city, on the other side of town.

"I sometimes would say to her, 'Why don't you get married so that I can have a brother or sister?' My mother never responded to the question. Her eyes would turn cold and she would leave the room.

"One Christmas after I moved to Canada, an aunt of mine, my mother's sister, was visiting. I guess it was by accident that she said something about my sister. I thought I had misheard. 'Your sister called me before I left last week,' she said.

"I walked right up to her and said, 'My sister?'

"And she covered her mouth with the palm of her right hand and whispered, 'Oh my god, you still don't know.' And like a spool of tightly wound yarn, the story of my parents and my sister unraveled itself on the living-room sofa.

"It was after that visit that I tried to make contact with my sister. It took me a year, and by that time, she was struggling with metastatic liver cancer and living in Hawaii. I sold my house to support her treatments and moved to Hawaii with her daughter. We stayed with my sister until she died, months later. That was five years ago. Now here I am with metastasized pancreatic cancer. And some people consider the pancreas to be the seat of nurturance and nutrition because it is connected to the gastrointestinal system.

"I've tried to talk to my mother. I'm sure her resistance is fortified by her guilt. She absolutely refuses to discuss it. She did not attend my sister's funeral. How is that for abandonment and betrayal? Why bring a child into the world and then reject it?"

The questions hang in the warm air of the group room. I unfold my legs.

Mothers and daughters. Daughters and mothers. Ritualized torture and execution. The uprising of the female Primal Horde. The ravishment of the Matriarch.

• • •

With my father, the lines of communication were direct, to the point.

"I like that dress." Period.

"I do not want you to date gentile boys." Period.

"I was brought up in an Orthodox home and I expect you to carry on with the same family traditions." Period.

Simple and direct. His words could be square or rectangular, but the lines were always neat and straight — no winding turns, no mazes, no ambiguities.

My mother, on the other hand, lived in a world of ambiguity. Words were camouflaged in hidden messages, in subterfuge and paradox.

"Mavis, I *really* like that pantsuit, but why don't you try on this one? The fabric is much nicer."

"It's not that I'm trying to interfere with your choices, *but* I think you would be better off without that friend of yours."

There were no limits, no boundaries for unsolicited advice. My mother had an opinion about everything: clothes, friends, dish detergents, furniture, nail polishes, relationships. Maternal prerogative (or was it imperative?), she called it.

"Just wait until you have children. You'll see what I mean. It's a mother's privilege to be honest with her daughter."

As I got older, I could not talk to my mother. Instead, I talked to my friends. My mother resented my friends, my social intimacies.

"Mavis, I am trying to talk to you," she would shout.

I stopped listening. I became untouchable. She wouldn't listen to me and I stopped paying attention to her. I barricaded myself in my room in the basement. I burned incense and listened to Bob Dylan and the Rolling Stones. But there was no lock on the door of the pink-and-peach bedroom. When my mother invaded my room, I traipsed off to the park, smoking cigarettes and reading Lawrence Ferlinghetti's *A Coney Island of the Mind*. I wrote poems of love and war. I lay on the grass and watched the constellations emerge against a blue-black sky. My parents thought I was turning into a hermit, or worse.

Years of arguments, impatient words, sullied moods, and abruptly ended conversations were to follow. A long process of "working through" would ensue. And then one day, the tension would dissolve and communication would resolve itself into two-way dialogue.

In university and in my ongoing studies I read about the mother-daughter relationship. Perhaps, like all daughters, I was searching for clues to my own inner turmoil. In my personal therapy, I spent hours hashing and rehashing the incidents, the moments marked by electric sparks and high voltage. I tried to understand the complexity of this bond.

Mothers. Rows of self-help books line the shelves of bookstores: books blaming mothers for their lack of attention, their narcissism, their impertinence and impotence, their abuse, their alcoholism, their mood disorders, their insecurities, their failed marriages . . . Daughters decrying their mothers for their mistakes, blaming them for their own unhappiness and failures, shunning them because of childhood pains and hardships . . . Mothers stalking the pages of novels and poems by Sylvia Plath, Anne Sexton, Adrienne Rich, Kim Chernin, Alice Walker. Images of mothers filling the pages of psychoanalytic literature: the phallic mother, the devouring mother, the primordial mother, the seductive mother . . .

The first truism: whatever the other differences, as human

beings we all share one thing in common — we are all born of a woman. Mothers are moored to the beginnings of life. The mother is the first love-object of the child.

As the primal source of life, the primary relationship after birth, mothers are easy targets. It is through the mother's eyes that the infant first perceives life. It is the mother who introduces the infant into the world of language by interpreting its screams and cries, thereby determining the first meanings of desire. It is the mother who soothes, bathes, feeds, satisfies, and frustrates the daughter in her early years. And it is from the mother that the daughter must transfer her loyalty and allegiance, first to her father and then to a partner.

From Greek mythology through the myths of Native Americans, from Old World to New World writings, the mother-daughter relationship has been central to women's life-struggle to free themselves from each other and to recognize each other as separate. Implicit in this painful separation is each woman's struggle to possess her own unencumbered truth — *her-story*. And yet it is exactly this psychological separation of mother and daughter that looms as "a paralysing threat over the life-land of the mother, and the future of the daughter." For many, these archaic formations lie suspended in the psyche, obstinately marking time. As Nini Herman writes,

> Here lies the world's greatest love affair, rapturous entanglement and deathtrap to development, in madness or in suicide; the wellspring of enduring strength or festering wound through which faint lives drain into oblivion. Only love on the grand scale, when it feels cheated or undone,

> can be subverted to the hatred where infanticide and matricide become ghostly denizens in that sun-drenched, golden land.

In his later years, Freud acknowledged that little girls have a strong attachment to their mothers that lasts for a lengthy period of time, predating the strong dependence on her father. What motivates the little girl to turn from her mother to her father? Freud writes,

> When we survey the whole range of motives for turning away from the mother — that she failed to provide the little girl with the only proper genital, that she did not feed her sufficiently, that she compelled her to share her mother's love with others, that she never fulfilled all the girl's expectations of love, and, finally, that she first aroused her sexual activity and then forbade it — all these motives seem nevertheless insufficient to justify the girl's final hostility. Some of them follow inevitably from the nature of infantile sexuality; others appear like rationalizations devised later to account for the uncomprehended change in feeling. Perhaps the real fact is that the attachment to the mother is bound to perish, precisely because it was the first and was so intense.

Is it that disappointments in early life are inevitable and, as they accumulate and multiply, so do the occasions for aggression and revenge? Is it the love affair with the father that forces the little girl to turn away from her first love-object, only to be rejected by him and thereby forced to leave him for another partner? Does the little girl then carry forward her turbulent feelings toward both parents into future adult relationships?

I am preparing my notes for an article, "Cancer and the Mother–Daughter Web." What happens to the mother–daughter bond when an already fragile family dynamic is exacerbated by a diagnosis of cancer? Thrown back into helplessness and a need for nurture originally supplied by the mother, tossed headlong into a state of flux, of personal re-evaluation, of reviewing life-narratives — is it surprising that old themes of mothers and daughters resurface?

The fact that this re-evaluation of family ties takes place under the strain of illness, and in some cases potential death, is bound to take its toll. For one thing, it encourages bringing up the most carefully concealed issues, anything to do with the family that is felt to be shameful: secrets, unforgivable acts, unresolved guilt, abandonment, and failures. On the other hand, a diagnosis of cancer may bring together a family that has been divided by rifts and resentments. In fighting a common goal, the family unit rallies in unity and bonds over its new objective, overlooking past hurts and betrayals.

And what about suspicions of a family curse, the possibility of a shortcoming in the genetic heritage? As the inheritor of a destructive gene from a mother who has cancer, a daughter may feel like the victim of a faulty family group. In turn, she may hate herself for her rage. At the same time, the mother may worry and feel guilty about her genetic makeup, feeling responsible for its impact on her children.

In the privacy of my office, I can deal with the particulars of each case. In the public forum, I am forced to make generalizations that dilute the facts of each family's uniqueness. I struggle with what to say about the issues of caretaking, involvement, and support. What is enough or too much? What is wanted or required? How do family members — mothers and daughters — begin to open the lines of communication for honest discussion, especially if no such precedent already exists?

And what about all the positive outcomes? What about all the instances where families *are* united and relationships cemented after years of battle, as physical vulnerability opens the door to acknowledgment of psychological vulnerability?

I open my pad and write: "In the midst of the emotional turmoil precipitated by a diagnosis of cancer, regressive patterns and archaic family dynamics once again become obvious . . ."

7

The fan is humming. Air circulates.

The women are seated in a circle — a circle of hope, of connection. These women are learning to bring hope to others. Harbingers of life. Themselves cancer survivors, they are learning to become peer-support counselors. Heroes. Stoics.

"Now I want you to think of ten things you can do for yourself that cost less than one dollar. Okay, maybe five dollars." Anne's voice swells across the room.

"How about a bubble bath?" someone calls out.

In the Peer Support Training session, we are talking about self-care. Care for the caregiver, learning to cope with stress and burnout. Anne's back is straight as she leans toward the flipchart and prints the words in bold letters: BUBBLE BATH.

"What else?" she asks the group. Anne is tall and thin. Her snow-white hair is brushed off her forehead. Her forehead is free of lines. Flat sandals, cotton pants, and a white shirt, a cardigan thrown over her shoulders. Anne looks tired today. The recent death of her granddaughter from a mysterious infection is taking its toll.

I had called Anne a week earlier. "Maybe it's too much for you to co-facilitate the training program now. Maybe you need a break," I suggested.

A pause from the other end, then a response, "You know what? It gets me out of myself and away from the pain. Let's do it together."

"If you're sure, that would be great," I said.

Anne brings the group back to the topic. This time, the voices compete to be heard: "A walk under the stars at night." "Blowing bubbles." "A meal cooked by your husband or a friend." "Coloring books."

"And how do you know you are stressed? How does your body tell you it is time to slow down?" Anne asks. She pauses a moment and then continues, "I know I am stressed when I get an ache in my shoulders."

Again the voices rise eagerly: "Headaches." "Can't get up in the morning." "Knots in my stomach." "Can't sleep." "Can't eat." "General body-ache." "I am quick to get a cold or flu."

"Yes," Anne responds. "The body signals like a telegraph, sending messages. It becomes important then to really listen to your body."

The two-day workshop draws to a conclusion. There have been tears and laughter. Members have been hurled into an experiential learning situation, with lectures on communication skills and definitions of peer support, role-play, and interactive teaching.

At the end, Anne leads the group through a closing exercise that reinforces hope and healing. Her voice is calm and even. "Let us all stand and hold hands . . . Imagine the light pouring down your hands, into your arms, spilling over into the center of the circle, so much light that you can draw energy and strength from it . . ."

After the training session, Anne and I meet with Holly, the new program director. We have both been drained by the demands of the workshop. We review concerns about particular individuals, glance through the evaluation forms, and debrief each other in terms of our reactions to the group.

"Sometimes I wonder how I do this, how I can keep coming back to this on beautiful weekends," Anne confesses, slouching back in her chair. "Yet it is such an important piece of our work."

"I sometimes wonder about the toll of this work on all of you leaders," Holly says.

"I know there are certainly times when I feel overwhelmed by it all," I add.

Anne speaks up. "We have to acknowledge our own human frailty. We don't like to, but we must. We so often confuse our roles as facilitator or therapist with our role as individuals who have the same problems as others. We do such a good job of keeping our place, our professional distance, that we are caught off guard when something happens in our personal lives. We almost believe that we are invincible because of our position in the group. That's nonsense. We are just as susceptible as anyone else to being diagnosed with an illness."

I am reminded of the family physician in my most recent group for metastatic disease. "My patients all told me that I was a doctor, I wasn't supposed to get sick," she had chuckled in the group. "Except, you know, I actually believed it, too."

"Maybe we need to have an informal buddy system for the professionals," Holly suggests.

"I think it happens informally anyway, the way Mavis and I speak to each other when we need to. I think it's already happening with the other group leaders."

"There is no magic in any of this," I say. "Last week in my young adult group, a member was talking about a friend who had relapsed. She said, 'I was stumped for words. I could only think I was glad it hadn't happened to me. Aren't I awful to think only of myself?' The rest of the members assured her that it was normal to feel that way. But they all agreed that it's difficult to come up with words of comfort in that situation. Yet sometimes I too feel it's a struggle to offer words of wisdom. I feel so impotent."

"Or is that our own belief, our own rescue fantasies at play?" counters Anne. "Sometimes, even we forget the power of listening — listening and hearing, listening without judging, without having to protect others, without having to keep up a brave pretense, without having to withhold tears. It's a pretty powerful tool."

I am often reminded of the truth of Anne's words when I sit listening, waiting for a patient to formulate a thought, to articulate an idea, to encounter something new that comes from deep within. The power of speaking from a place of truth.

Holly gets ready to leave, gathering her briefcase and handbag. "Thanks again for the great day. Just make sure you lock up when you leave."

Anne and I don't move. I have grown to trust Anne. She is my senior in years, and I look to her as a mentor. As someone who has had breast cancer herself, she understands the issues from both sides, as a patient and as a professional. It is to Anne that I turn when I need to talk about difficulties I am experiencing with listening, with hearing, with despair. It is to Anne that I turn when I question what we can offer to others when it all seems so bleak and somber.

She says thoughtfully, "You know, we really don't take this stuff seriously enough. We keep encouraging our patients to be attuned to the signs and signals of burnout. We keep encouraging peer-support volunteers at Wellspring to listen to their bodies and make time to relax, to look after themselves so they won't become tired or burned out. Yet here we are, confronted almost daily with the constancy, the tenacity, the terror of cancer, and we ignore these lessons ourselves."

"Absolutely true. It's always listening to stories of chaos, of pain and suffering, of family breakdown, of financial crisis and mental dysfunction. It's like a simmering pot about to boil over."

"And how big are your rescue fantasies these days? Mine are diminishing daily with my granddaughter's death."

"We really are good actresses, you know. You too," I laugh, nudging her arm. "We hide our vulnerabilities from the group and stay firm in our position."

"You mean I'm *allowed* to feel something, like really be human?" Anne jokes, as we both get up. "Right."

"But we both know that's what it's about. If we stop feeling anything, we're dead. We stop being able to do this work."

"I'm just teasing you, Mavis. You're right. It's about balancing our ability to acknowledge our feelings without being so overwhelmed that we can't do it anymore."

"I don't know about you, but I'm wiped out."

"Let's get out of here — fast."

Anne and I turn out the lights, lock up, and once again embrace. The rituals of working together. The bonds of friendship.

• • •

Lydia tells me that I must slow down my pace. She points at me with her manicured finger and says, "Your shoulders, kid. They are definitely growing humps."

The eucalyptus steam room at Ste. Anne's Country Inn and Spa is a welcome relief after the low-impact cardio workout.

"Your eyes are beginning to droop," Lydia continues.

"Just what I need to hear. I suppose everything else on my body will be drooping, too, in a couple of years." I look up at Lydia's small frame perched on the teak bench above me. I remember that she once considered breast enlargement to enhance her "feminine charm" after her ex-boyfriend accused her of having miniature breasts. "Go to hell," she had said to him, and then spent the next three months trying to pull herself back together again.

"It feels as though the force of gravity is starting to work on me — sagging breasts, sagging jowls, sagging buttocks, and flat feet. You should be thankful for those 'miniatures.'"

Lydia laughs. "Do we ever give up? When do we stop kidding

ourselves about the inevitability of A-G-E?"

"My mother just turned seventy-five and she says she is still fighting it. Just hit me with some reality testing if I start taking belly-dancing classes or chasing some twenty-year-old when I'm in my sixties."

I have known Lydia for over twenty years. We met when our cars gently kissed in a parking lot; since then, we have become close friends. Lydia is a social worker for a children's mental health center. Her compact size is a paradox to her co-workers, who think of her as larger than life. She has a loud, powerful voice, and she likes to speak out on the dangers of chronic burnout in professionals. Her work with battered women and children has made her immune to a system that rewards unrealistic caseloads and unremitting piles of paperwork.

Visible scars, invisible scars. Unlike cancer patients, the abused women do not suffer from surgical mutilation or genetic mutations. Instead their bodies bear the marks of intentional pain, hidden bruises, memories that cannot be erased. These women do not know about self-worth. Their bodies are objects of torment, not desire.

Lydia pours some water onto the pile of stones and a mist of fresh steam sizzles into the enclosed space. We settle into a companionable silence . . .

Suddenly, I feel a light touch on my arm. Someone is whispering my name. "Mavis, we've been here for over fifteen minutes. I think we're scheduled for a seaweed body wrap. And our bodies are turning into prunes." We slide off the wooden benches and swaddle our heated bodies in scented terry kimonos.

A woman in a white smock invites me into the massage room and introduces herself as Maria. She asks me to get on the table, and I slide under the sheet, my body still warm from the body mask treatment. She asks me a few questions about my general health and any physical problems and then slowly begins to work on my back.

"You have tense shoulders," Maria says, massaging my neck and upper arms. I am on my stomach on a cushioned cot, my face cupped in a sling. I attempt to respond, but my feeble grunts of agreement fall to the floor below.

Her touch is penetrating, yet gentle. Maria's fingers feel long, her hands masculine in their strength. She leans into my natural rhythms and my body purrs in contentment. Maria reminds me of my grandmother, full-bodied and curvaceous. Like my grandmother, she is also East European. I ask her where she is from.

"I am from Czechoslovakia. Only here four months."

I ask her about her perceptions of Canada.

"Here, there is much to enjoy. Back home, there is more politics than TV. But since I leave, my parents get more food in the lineups. Is better now."

I ask why she moved to Canada, hoping that my question will not offend her.

She responds in clipped tones. "Everyone in America think that people want to come here because life is better, more money here. Is not true. Only those already with money can come. People here do not understand Europe — my part of Europe."

I drift away from the talk and allow myself to be transported by the sounds of a tape of wind chimes and harp. Maria works her confident way around my body, kneading all the muscle groups I have heard about in my fitness classes. When she is done, she says, "You can rest here until you ready. It is good to lie for five, ten minutes."

With the second day at Ste. Anne's still ahead of us, time begins to slow down. Lydia and I decide to go for a walk after our lunch of local mineral water, Waldorf salad with raspberry vinaigrette, and a cheese plate. We fill our water bottles and set out down the road. On all sides we are surrounded by a patchwork quilt of brown and green fields — cornstalks, wheat, hay, soybeans.

An open truck passes us, swirling dust up to our waists. Three tanned girls with sun-bleached pigtails and baseball caps wave, their giggles trailing behind in the wind.

"Listen to that sound," I say, a few minutes later. "There's water nearby." But then I look up and see the poplar leaves rustling; I know that nature has once again deceived me. I hear Lawlor's voice whispering, "They always sound like waterfalls in the wind."

As you climb Academy Hill Road, you come to a cemetery sitting at the top of the hill. Continuing along the road, you reach a stone wall that encloses a fortress-like castle. This is your initial impression when you arrive at Ste. Anne's, the site of rest, relaxation, and rejuvenation.

According to local lore, the Massey family settled in a log house in this Northumberland County valley in the early 1800s. In 1836 two of the sons each built themselves a stone house on opposite hilltops in order to oversee the old homestead. The homes were identical, their walls three feet thick. One house is currently owned by a retired Toronto physician and the other by the Corcoran family, who transformed their home into Ste. Anne's.

Their brochure proudly announces that, in addition to the castle with its ten guest rooms and spa facilities, five off-site houses are scattered among the hills of Northumberland. The spa packages have names like Strength after Struggle, Quiet Reflection, and Primal Elements for Men, suggesting the broad array of available activities. Body-work, aesthetic treatments, hydrotherapy, and heat treatments have all contributed to Ste. Anne's popularity.

As we veer off onto a country side road, Lydia begins to tell me about a difficult case that is challenging her. "This woman was so close to being permanently brain-injured by her husband, according to the emergency doc. And she insists that his 'little outburst' was justified because his supper was burnt for the second day in a row. Give me a break! And her son is turning into a carbon copy of his father."

"Good luck. I don't know how you do that work."

"Me? What about you? I'd like to know how you do all that work with sick and dying people. What keeps you going back?"

"You know, once I met a Greek man in Mexico — shipping magnate, well turned-out, white hair, distinguished gait. I had been traveling by myself and he was friendly, inquisitive, almost seductive. He asked me what I did in my spare time and I decided to shock him. So I said, 'I help the dying.' And he said, 'You've got to be joking.' Then I came back with, 'It's punishment for all my sins.' Man, did that ever keep him quiet!"

"No, I mean it. What drives you?"

"No shop talk, I thought we said."

"This isn't shop talk. This is philosophy. Don't you ever get depressed from all of that cancer? Doesn't it get to you? Doesn't it distort your view of the world? I would probably be a mess after a few months of it."

"I don't know. It's such powerful and meaningful work that, in some strange way, I find it very rewarding. In the groups, I don't do anything. I know that I have no secret potion to take away the cancer, to remove the malignant cells. There's no magic cure for pain and suffering. I can accept that. I can accept that what I have to offer is something else. So, no, it doesn't depress me or destroy my passion for life. Maybe it's the opposite. I mean, maybe it's what I learn from them, from all those cancer patients. The gift is being able to see the world through their perspective without the torture of the diagnosis. It's like I'm able to appreciate what I've got and keep my perspective when I start bitching about the small stuff. Does that make sense to you?"

"Yes, absolutely. I get what you mean. But it still seems depressing to me."

"I never said I don't get depressed at times or that it never gets me down. Of course I have my moments, my days. But I also have a deep belief in the value of this kind of work, in being able to provide a safe place for people to share their fears and anxieties about death, about sexuality, about everything. And, I suppose, it's also what I am able to give of myself in order to help people who are struggling with questions of pain and mortality and meaning."

That night I lay awake ruminating about Lydia's question. How many times have I asked myself why I do this work in spite of the emotional toll it takes? How do I recharge my own batteries? Where does my desire to pursue this work come from?

I enter into relationships with strangers who are suffering from a terrifying disease. I become briefly involved in their lives. I listen to their pain, their fears. I know from the start that death is a persistent reality. And yet there is the other side as well. I am bolstered by the strength, determination, and vitality of the human spirit in the face of cancer. I am touched and moved by the honesty and virtue of the words. I am able to share in the humor and laughter of so many wonderful men and women.

I know this work is in some ways connected to my genetic inheritance. For me, my biological destiny on my maternal side is definitely under the sign of the Crab. Perhaps by plunging myself into the world of oncological research I am learning about my inheritance, arming myself with an imaginary arsenal of words, seeking a protective shield of information, uncovering new weapons of treatment.

And my unconscious anxieties? I know less about those. Perhaps I too am able to work through the fears of mortality, of loss, of the unknown. I know that when my sister was diagnosed with cancer — the first of my generation — I was plagued by a deep dread. I too felt that I could no longer parade and masquerade and sleepwalk through life. I too felt that I would have to confront my demons head-on.

The gift in it for me? In the groups I learn by osmosis the value of my strong limbs, my pumping heart, my clear lungs. I am grateful for my well-functioning body. It is certainly a gift to be able to learn the value of life without being diagnosed with cancer.

I do not offer prayers of thanks through institutionalized religion. Perhaps I should, but it is not my way. Instead I push and pull and stretch my limbs. I hike and bike and paddle and jump and dance and climb and swim. I do not take for granted this assembly of bones, muscles, tendons, and tissues that I call my physical self. I push its limits to remind myself that I am alive.

When I lived in Israel, I would pack a small knapsack of essentials: canvas boots, red-topped army socks, T-shirt, sweater, a package of sunflower seeds, two cans of hummus, two packages of pita, orange and yellow cheese, *wafflim* cookies, and a canteen. I would catch the last bus out of Tel Aviv on Friday afternoon and make my way to the meeting site where a group of like-minded hikers from the Society for the Preservation of Nature gathered. Every weekend I was introduced to a new landscape of this miniature country: Nahal Bezet, Ein Qilt, Berekhat Ram, Beit She'arim, Tel Hai, Har Tabor. Water sites, hills, deserts, seashores, valleys, caves.

Some voice beckoned me to the land around, this precious land threatened by external enemies. Here I could flex my muscles, lose myself in the energy of the day's activities, and fall asleep exhausted. Here, by the jagged cliffs or silky sands or blue waters in a homeland of wanderers, I could feel myself at peace in the universe and give thanks for the intact landscape of my sacred body.

• • •

"The benefits of cancer . . . You know, there are some. I'm embarrassed to say that and I would only say it in this room," Tove says, staring at her boots. She lifts her head and continues,

"We have to be honest here, don't we?"

Preeya is curled under a blanket and looks tired. Lily and Carole nod their heads in agreement.

"I know, it's easy to fall into a victim mentality. 'Poor me, I've got cancer. Feel sorry for me,'" Lily says.

"Is that what you mean?" Carole asks.

"Oh, yes, for sure. But I was thinking of benefits in even more subtle ways. Like going to visit my mother. You know I wrote her and asked if she would consider not smoking for the week when I visit her at Christmas. I said it was for medical reasons, without mentioning my diagnosis. This week she wrote back that it would not be convenient for her. I got the message all right — she prefers smoking to seeing her daughter . . ."

Gasps of disgust, head-shaking, heavy sighs.

"Well," Tove continues, "I wanted to pick up the phone and call Denmark and shout in her ear, 'I'm dying of cancer and you may never see me again, so I hope you can live with that, you stupid old woman!' I even dreamed of visiting her at my funeral and tapping her on the shoulder, saying, 'It's all your fault; you could have prevented it.'"

I am not sure how the group will respond to Tove's honesty. I hold my breath and wait.

"You're right, Tove. Sometimes I want to say to someone in the bank line, 'Let me ahead of you, I have less time than you. I'm dying of cancer.' Or 'Feel sorry for me, I'm in such pain,'" Carole picks up.

"And yet," the reasonable calm of Lily interrupts, "isn't there the other benefit? The one about appreciating life? I find that everything has a heightened intensity about it. I celebrate

Thanksgiving; I invite my friends and we prepare a veritable feast and I eat what I can because — who knows? — it might be the last. Or I stand looking at the rose beds in Edwards Gardens, and I really do see something else, something so magnificent it makes me cry."

I remember Nathalie, from a previous group, saying, "I had wanted something in my life to change, to help me change, but I sure didn't need to be hit over the head with a sledgehammer."

And I remember Mary from the same group: "Well, if it was a choice between *not* smelling the roses or a diagnosis of cancer, I think I'd pass up the damn roses and the reflection of trees in the water and the rest of it. That's just a bunch of bullshit created by others to try and make us feel good."

The other members shifted in their chairs, but let her outburst slip by without comment. Yet it was Mary, eight days before her death, who was transported by her closest friends to a lake by the family cottage and dipped in the water as if for baptism.

And I remember reading Rachel Naomi Remen, medical director of the Commonweal Cancer Help program in Bolinas, California, who said, "I really worry about people who get cancer and don't get angry, because I feel that somehow they're not holding to life, they're not engaged with life, or they're not passionate enough about life. . . . Anger is a demand for change."

The group seems refreshed this week. There is an energy that was absent last time we met.

"I want to go back to that question," I say. "What about the benefits? We never got to that last week."

Each of the members responds in turn.

Carole: "It's that cliché, the 'wake-up call.' I've had to learn to get my priorities straight. It's not how I wanted to be shocked, but it is a force to reckon with."

Preeya: "Like taking stock. I appreciate what I have: my husband, my daughter, my church, my friends."

Tove: "It's forced me to come to peace quickly with a lot of unfinished business. If I don't have a lot of time left, then I want to leave this world without any dirty laundry. I want to be remembered with the respect and honor I am owed. As difficult as this is, I am trying to forgive her — my mother — even though she doesn't think she needs forgiveness."

Carole: "I just picked up this new book by Stephen Levine, called *A Year to Live*. He says that it is important to go through the process of 'affirmation, forgiveness and acceptance.' It's sure not easy when your family keeps avoiding you or fighting with you."

Tove: "But I look at it this way: maybe that's the best they can do right now. If I can set an example by not getting caught up in their issues, I preserve my energy for other things."

Lily: "I remember my husband saying to me once, 'You just have to take care of yourself. You got nothing to do with them neighbors who just like to gossip all day. They gonna talk, talk, talk, whether you nice or not. So you just get on with your living.'"

Preeya: "I try to take walks when I'm upset. It's getting harder now, with my legs getting weaker. And I'm beginning to have odd sensations and fatigue in my arms. I have an appointment with the neurologist on Friday. My oncologist thinks there may be something else going on."

Tove: "Is this the doctor who's been avoiding your calls?"

Preeya: "Yes, but lately she's been returning my calls on the same day."

And the conversation moves in and out of changes in life, in lifestyle, in living — and continues.

Carole: "I do find myself returning to that question 'Why me?' Not in an angry, resentful way, more in terms of 'What am I supposed to learn from this?'"

Lily: "You mean 'What is the message?'"

Carole: "Yes. How do I make sense of this diagnosis, this cancer? What does it mean in my life? How can I turn it into a positive? Remember that other book, the one by the psychologist Lawrence LeShan? He talked about that. I'm still trying to figure it all out. The problem is, I thought I had it all figured out the first time around, fifteen years ago. I could slow down, enjoy what I had. But now, with this metastatic stuff, I'm losing strength. I don't know anymore. I can't come up with any answers, and my family thinks I'm giving up."

Lily: "But Carole, look at you. You are such a fighter. I look at you and you're a role model for me. Here you are, ten years later, when they said you had six months. Different treatments, and you're still here, honey."

Tove: "How could anyone say you're a quitter? You've been putting up with one chemo after another for years. No way you're a quitter! None of us are, or we wouldn't be here."

The session continues to unfold. I follow the conversation back and forth across the room — a tapestry of interwoven threads.

8

Diana died on July 14. Mona died on July 23. Nicholas died on August 4. Harry died on August 11. Erica died on August 25. I write down the names and dates so I won't forget. I repeat the words to myself. Rehearsing. Does repetition ease the pain, obliterate the memories?

Some of the women are already seated. I gather my notes and prepare a cup of Cozy Camomile tea. Terry greets me with a warm hug. It's after the summer break, and I notice that her hair has grown back and she is no longer wearing a hat. Selma, Nathalie, and Louise arrive at the same time, breathless from the late summer heat. They each collapse into a chair. Peggy's salt-and-pepper hair is curly from the humidity and her skin glistens.

Nathalie has gained weight and walks with a limp. Choruses of greetings sing through the room.

"How was your summer?"

"Good. I was at the cottage. And what about you?"

"Ongoing chemo. No holiday from the ward."

"Don't you look great! Look at your hair."

I bring the group to attention and place five green candles on the coffee table. Everyone is instantly solemn and attentive. I wait until the introductory visualization exercise is over before I address the candles. Diana died on July 14, Mona died on July 23, Nicholas died on August 4, Harry died on August 11, Erica died on August 25. The words shatter the silence.

I invite a different member to light each of the candles. One by one, they are placed in the glass bowl of water.

I study my knees momentarily. Black stockings. Catch near the knee — should have changed them.

I tell the group what I have been told by relatives, friends. My voice flattens into a monotone. Diana was at home; her best friend Reena was with her, as well as her brother; she was comfortable, not in pain, and drifted out in a semi-coma. Mona was at the Grace in the palliative unit; her family was with her a few hours before she died; she told the nurse about her group at Wellspring and how she would miss everyone.

I hear sniffling and the rustling sound of tissues. I feel my voice cracking as I continue, "I have no information about Harry, as I was not in touch with him or his wife after he stopped attending the group. And Nicholas did manage to go up to his cottage for most of the summer with his fiancée. They had a great time and then they returned home when Nick began to feel sicker. I talked to him a week before he died and he sounded very peaceful. He said that he knew he had little time left, but he wanted you all to know how much the group meant to him."

Terry is the first to speak, blowing her nose intermittently. "It's no fair . . . It's just no fair. But . . . I went to Mona's funeral. I was in touch with her a few days before she died. I had to go to the funeral, even though I didn't know a soul. I felt very displaced. But I want to tell you what her husband and parents said. When they found out who I was and that I was from her support group, they hugged me and said, 'You probably knew her best of all. She always spoke about her group at Wellspring.'"

Terry stopped, sighed, and continued. This time her words were measured and slow. "I want you all to know my husband, so I brought in a picture of him. If I die . . . and I know I will one day, then I want you all to feel comfortable enough to attend my funeral. So I'm going to circulate this photo. Here."

Terry holds the picture out to Nathalie and it circulates around the circle. Then her round face opens momentarily in a broad grin as she chides herself, "Not like I want to get maudlin or anything on you guys."

Nathalie's shoulders are shaking. "Diana, Diana," she mutters in a semi-whisper. "I talked to her three nights before she died. We have the same diagnosis. I can't believe it. Her friend — remember Reena? She used to always mention her. Well, Reena called me the next day and told me there would be a small memorial service at the end of the month."

My mouth is parched. Words fall in dry showers.

"Look, I think we need to be there for each other at the end. We've all agreed on that." I do not see who is speaking.

"Yet how realistic is it? When Sheila died, her son and daughter were with her, and with Harold, it was his wife. Yet we all say that we will be there for each other."

Sarah's mass of blonde curls bobs up and down as she nods in agreement.

"We can be there if it works out that way. You are all my biggest support. I do want you to be there at the end. But if that doesn't happen, then I'll still know how important you all are to me," Pat says.

"You know, this is hell, all these deaths, all this . . ." Selma waves her hands in frustration. "Yet somehow I would rather be here than not be here. My husband thinks I'm crazy. He sometimes says, 'Why go if you sometimes feel worse after?' And I simply say, 'It's my support, and I have to go.'"

• • •

My sister, Linda, and I shared a bedroom. Lying on our smooth pink sheets, we would taunt each other with ghoulish questions as we pondered the mysteries of life and death. What do you think happens when you die? Can you imagine being dead and the world going on and on and on without you?

Linda would return to that question with the irritating regularity of a refrain. I, on the other hand, would pull the pillow over my head in order to blot out the macabre images.

As a child, I certainly did not know what happened after you died, at least not in the metaphysical or theological sense. I only knew that the body was placed in a casket that was buried in the ground and that there was a ritual at the cemetery to mark this passage.

When my grandfather died, I was eight years old. I knew that he was ill with something called leukemia. My mother would drive back and forth between the hospital and my grandparents' apartment. She would return home late at night, her face red and puffy. My father would warn us that my mother was tired, and not to bother her with too many questions. Then, on a blustery, cold day in January, my mother came home from the hospital and announced that Zaide had died. My sister began to laugh. I ran up to my room and buried my head in a pillow.

The day of my grandfather's funeral, my mother wore a black skirt with a charcoal-gray sweater and black pumps. I thought she looked ugly, but I did not want to tell her because she had already been crying that morning. I was not allowed to go to the funeral service or the cemetery. Linda and I had to stay home with Ninetta, the cleaning lady, who usually came only on Mondays. We helped Ninetta cut up pieces of honey cake and place sliced bagels on a platter with lox and cream cheese.

"People will be hungry. Is so sad, so sad. Must make it all look nice like your mother likes it," Ninetta said, as if having a conversation with herself. I did not understand why she was so sad when she did not know my zaide.

The mirrors in the house were draped with white sheets and pillowcases, the doorbell was covered with tape, and a pitcher of water was placed outside. I thought my mother would be mad at Ninetta for putting it on the special china plate with pink-and-white magnolias. When my parents and grandmother returned from the funeral, they poured water from the pitcher over their hands and chanted some words in Hebrew. My mother's face was splotchy and she held on to my grandmother's arm. My grandmother was in the black taffeta dress that she wore only on special occasions. Her face was vacant, as if all expression had been rubbed out.

Within minutes of their arrival, I noticed a parade of cars that stopped to park along the crowded street. A stream of people — my parents' friends, second and third cousins with unfamiliar names and faces — made their way to the front door, each taking a turn with the china jug. Some of the women carried trays of Danish pastries, coffeecake, and more bagels.

Inside the house, Ninetta was frantically trying to find appropriate serving dishes. "It's okay, Ninetta," my Auntie Jean kept repeating. "Just use whatever there is."

"But Mrs. 'imes, you know, she is very fussy lady," Ninetta insisted. "She like things in special way. I no want Mrs. 'imes be mad at me."

"It's okay, Ninetta. For today, it's all right to use anything." Auntie Jean took it upon herself to rummage through cupboards of neatly assembled plates and bowls and trays in lacquered papier-mâché, Italian gold leaf, and laminated plastic until she found some platters with green and yellow borders.

Many people came and went through the house that day and in the days to follow. My grandmother slept on the extra bed in the guest room. She asked to borrow my pillow, and I felt that I was contributing in some significant way to a special cause and that God would reward me for the sacrifice. My grandmother spent the entire week at our house. Within months she had moved into the carpeted room at the bottom of the stairs. Sometimes I would hear her sniffling in her bed.

• • •

Children think about death the way they think about the rest of life's mysteries, from clouds and rainbows, leaping frogs and falling leaves, to unicorns and flying pterodactyls. In the world of boys and girls, life takes on an intensity of color and meaning that is built up from a need to create order out of chaos.

Richard Lonetto, a psychologist who studied children's conceptions of death, once asked school-aged children to describe and discuss their drawings of death. He found that children attempt to create an integrated world that encompasses both life and death. Only later, after they have established a sense of time and causality, do they superimpose more abstract concepts on the earlier, immature ones. According to Lonetto, it is as if we know as children about the experience of oneness, forget about it as we grow, and then spend a lifetime trying to recreate the blissfulness of unity.

When I thought about death as a young child, I imagined an underground world where people ate rotten food on splintered plates and sat on dwarfed chairs with wobbly legs. Later I modified my view, imagining the earth opening up and consuming your body while the mind continued to live on, active and restless. I imagined that when you were buried, you could not touch the hand of your neighbor, that you were cut off and isolated. The underground world of death was a terrifying abyss.

When I gave workshops on bereavement for children, I would also ask them to draw pictures of death. "If you could draw a picture of death, what would it look like?" I asked the different age groups. They produced monsters and scary-looking giants; they created caricatures of evil-looking sorcerers, ghosts, graves, and cemeteries; they filled pages with black scribbles and geometric columns, small-scale worlds peopled by stunted creatures.

These artworks confirmed what the reference books indicated. Preschoolers do not have a grasp of the permanence of death. For them, death is a place like life, filled with restaurants and theaters, milkshakes and ice cream cones, Tarzan and Batman, mommies and daddies and unwanted teachers. It is when children become school-aged that death becomes an external agent that can snatch you and take you away — a ghost, a five-headed monster, a black blob, an invisible force that can steal boys and girls in the night. Later, these personifications become transformed into the more adult standard, where death is perceived as the end of life — final, painful, the Great Blackness.

My image of death as an underground tunnel stayed with me for many years. I would lie in bed, shivering with cold as I responded to my sister's insistent questions. I imagined myself buried alive, suffocating and unable to reach another human being. When my father died, that image returned to haunt me.

• • •

At the beginning of the fast of Tishah B'Av, which marks the destruction of the first temple in 586 BCE by Nebuchadnezzar and of the second temple in 70 CE by the Romans, traditional mourners eat eggs and bread dipped in ashes while sitting on a hard floor. An egg is also eaten at the completion of the fast. It is believed in the Jewish tradition that because the egg is round and contains no opening, it symbolizes life.

At my grandmother's funeral, a bowl of hard-boiled eggs sits regally in a glass bowl in the middle of the dining-room table. A white linen tablecloth, embroidered by my grandmother as a young woman, lies across the table. Crease marks, humped in equidistant rectangles, expose the folds of age. Was it my grandmother herself who last ironed the cloth?

I am no longer a child. I help lay out the platters of honey cake and coffeecake, the settings of teacups and coffee spoons, and the gold-trimmed plates used for special occasions. My mother insists that there be smoked salmon, bagels, and cream cheese. "No one should think we're scrimping," she mutters under her breath.

My father nods in agreement, too tired to argue about principles. "Yes, dear. We will have everything in order."

There is one low wooden chair in the den — for the only daughter, the only survivor of her family. One chair, one candle, one mother, one father, one daughter. One God of Judaism. Unity — unity in fragmentation.

My mother will sit on the low wooden chair for seven days. She will rise only for meals and for sleep. She will not be forced to say Kaddish. Three times a day, a *minyan* of ten men will gather to recite prayers.

One woman. She will not be counted among the ten. One daughter equals no voice. My mother is an egg — mute.

I hear the words of the mourners downstairs, muffled sounds of chanting. The words of the mourners' Kaddish carry through the house: *Yit'gadal v'yit'kadash sh'may rabba . . .* From the top of the landing, I see the figures of fifteen men sway back and forth. Long prayer shawls cover their shoulders. One of the men has also covered his head.

As I look down from the landing, I can see my father in his

prayer shawl. His white hair lies flat against his forehead. A handsome man, my father.

Tzefat, also known as Safed — the city of mysticism, one of the sacred cities of Israel's history. Tzefat reached the height of its fame in the sixteenth century, when Kabbalists flocked to it from exile and converted it into a city of mystic lore. Buried near Tzefat is the body of Rabbi Shimon Bar Yochai, to whom is attributed the *Zohar* ("splendor"), the fundamental work of the Kabbalah, which is also referred to as *Hochma Nisteret,* the Secret Wisdom. The mystics believed that the air of Tzefat, which is about 900 meters above sea level on Mount Canaan, was the purest air of the Holy Land, and inspirational for understanding the profundities of the Holy Torah.

Today the main street of Tzefat, Rechov Yerushalayim (Jerusalem Road), encircles the mountain and is the main traffic artery. I walk down from this main street into a series of crooked lanes and cobbled stone streets. I stroll into all the famous ancient synagogues: the Ha'ari Synagogue of the Ashkenazim; the Bana'a Synagogue; the Ha'ari Synagogue of the Sephardim; Chakal Tapuchim ("Field of Apples"), its poetic name designating paradise in the mystical tradition. I am overwhelmed by the beauty and simplicity of these houses of worship.

Off a cobblestone street in the artists' colony, I enter a damp, dark shop. Candelabra, menorahs, tefillin, mezuzahs — Judaica and religious artifacts clad in silver and pewter, brass and ceramic — crowd every niche. A short man, hunched apparently by years of prayer, welcomes me. "*Shalom, shalom. Boi, boi* [Come in, come in]."

In the old-fashioned Ashkenazi accent of my father, grandfather, and great-grandfather, he invites me to look around, take my time, not to rush — just enjoy the beauty of these holy artifacts. He returns to his stool and continues polishing a silver goblet.

A smell of holiness. What does holiness smell like?

I decide to buy a prayer shawl for my father, a *tallit*. I select one in a delicate fabric with a blue pattern, and add a purple velvet carrying case. Then I add a *kippah*, a royal-blue velvet skullcap with silver embroidery. The bright color will highlight his white hair.

The shopkeeper — his name is Hymie, I learn, the same as my maternal grandfather — is pleased with my purchases. I tell him the gifts are for my father. I tell him that I come from Montreal, Canada, and that I am presently living in Rechovot. I tell him these things in his own language so that I can feel a sense of connection, of ethnic community with this septuagenarian who looks at me through thick bifocals.

"Oy, Canada," he says. "I have a cousin in Canada, a third cousin on my sister's side." And without pausing, he asks me if I might know his cousin, his name is Asher, Asher Horowitz, and he teaches Hebrew. He teaches young children in a cheder.

"You must know a cheder in the old section of Montreal," he says, "where all the *yidlich* live." As he speaks, he folds the *tallit* and *kippah* into a small square, his fingers stroking the fabric intimately. Then he wraps them delicately in brown paper.

"Because you are from Canada, I will give you a special price," he says, and I smile inwardly.

I no longer remember how many shekels he discounted or

even whether there were price tags attached to the articles. I paid him and he shook my hand.

"*A shaina tochter. Zei guezunt* [A nice daughter. Be well]," I heard him say as I closed the door behind me.

• • •

My doctoral thesis supervisor at the University of Toronto, Glenn MacDonald, reminded me of a teddy bear. He looked as though he hadn't grown into his skin, which pleated around his neck and his wrists. I always thought of him as older than his years, because of his thinning brandy-colored hair. He had thin lips that were usually pinched shut. With his dry, sardonic wit and expressionless face, it was hard to tell whether he was laughing to himself or with you.

Glenn was my supervisor for my Master's thesis in psychology. I asked him to supervise me again when I returned to university two years later to complete my doctoral degree.

Six foot two, eyes of blue. Glenn was the image of a professor in his gray flannels with the baggy cuffs that dragged over his Hush Puppies. In winter he wrapped a long burgundy scarf around his neck. He once told me that his wife had knitted him the scarf, so he felt obliged to show his appreciation by wearing it, even though he disliked the color. That was the most personal statement Glenn ever made to me.

For my doctoral dissertation I decided to study beginnings — the beginnings of language development. I observed the motion, commotion, and locomotion between mothers and their toddlers while I recorded the speech patterns of both. In a softly lit room emptied of distractions, I watched mothers and infants play with a cuddly brown bear, a book, a ball. I hid behind the clumsy recording equipment and filmed my subjects. I coded their conversations and learned that language learning and language teaching are entwined in a web of interactive mutuality.

When I was a year into my research, Glenn was diagnosed with non-Hodgkin's lymphoma. Over the next few months he lost weight, his hair, and his humor. Life was squeezed into the spaces between his treatments. And then, as if by a miracle, his hair grew back, his body resumed its old shape, and the jokes percolated to the surface once more.

In the meantime, my research was taking shape. I was videotaping mothers and infants, chauffeuring them back and forth in my military-green Datsun to an old brick house in the university annex. The preliminary results looked promising, and I was about to begin the arduous task of statistical analysis.

As rapid as his initial recovery was Glenn's relapse and subsequent deterioration. He was once again admitted to the hospital. His vitality dwindled, eroded by the onslaught of malignant cell activity. I began to visit him at the hospital. We talked about horse races and football. I brought him an apple-spice loaf I had baked from a recipe that I had carefully copied from one of my mother's cookbooks. He was not able to eat even that.

Glenn wished me well on my departmental orals. He was too ill to attend. "You can fool them on those statistics. Just sock it to them. You have nothing to worry about," he said, coughing out a laugh.

My knees shook as I stood outside the university lecture room where I was to be interrogated for my thesis defense. The other committee members smiled, only feigning support. The external examiners were well rehearsed. I answered all the questions.

Glenn died two weeks before my senate orals. At the funeral there was a guitarist who wore an Indian sari and African buffalo sandals. Her hair was long and shone in the sunlight. She sang "We Shall Overcome" on the lawn outside the church. A crowd of people piled inside for the service that followed. That night I got drunk.

• • •

November 1998. My neighbor is dying of cancer. He is lying at home in a hospital bed, propped up on an air mattress, supported by machines that pump the bare essentials into his feeble body. Five months ago, Scott surprised his wife, Carrie, by taking her on an anniversary trip to Holland and France. Four months ago, Scott participated in a fundraising run. On the August long weekend, Scott was diagnosed with metastatic cancer. His body was riddled with disease; both lungs were full of tumors.

When Carrie first told me, poking her head through the overgrown bushes, she just shook her head. "His lungs look like those of a sixty-five-year-old who's been smoking two packs a day for forty years. How can that be? He never touched a cigarette in his life."

I could feel my eyes widen and grow moist as I squinted behind my sunglasses. "What do they say, the doctors?"

"Unknown primary, metastasized to the bones, lungs, lymph nodes, and possibly liver. The good news is that there was an elevated blood count in his prostate, so they're checking that out as a possibility. In the meantime, it's tests, tests, and more tests until they can determine the primary. And a ton of radiation to his spine to ease the pain." Carrie spoke without affect.

I checked my encyclopedia on cancer therapy. Primary prostate cancer: good prognosis, curable. Primary lung cancer with metastatic disease: not good prognosis, five-year survival less than five percent. Who consults encyclopedias? Who believes in statistics anymore?

A few days later, the test results eliminated prostate cancer and Scott was diagnosed as having a rare type of squamous-cell lung cancer. Chemotherapy was attempted. Radiation therapy shrank the tumors in his back but could not eliminate the debilitating pain as they kept appearing like popcorn on his spine.

In the first few weeks after the diagnosis, Scott and Carrie arranged their schedule like honeymooners. Every week they attempted to head up north to the family cottage on Lake Muskoka. "You should see the colors — so amazing," Scott said one evening when they returned. "The peak of fall's splendor."

"Sounds great," I said.

"The evenings are a bit brisk, but it's so peaceful up there. I sleep a lot from my chemo and this damn thing," Scott said, tugging on his portable morphine pump.

He had lost most of his thick blond hair, but his blue eyes were still radiant. "You know what?" he continued. "This cancer's a mysterious thing. We feel we can fight it. If it came so suddenly and mysteriously, then it may leave in the same way. We've got to remain optimistic, Carrie and I. We can't let this get us down. I'm young and healthy. I know I can beat this thing."

I began praying that night. Praying that Scott would live to share those words with his future children. Praying that Emma and Paula, Tom and Kevin, Frank and Elizabeth, and all the other young people whom I knew would survive their disease and outlive their prognoses of premature death. I sat in the beige chair in Lawlor's study and stared at the Buddha with his fat, healthy belly, wondering what made sense.

A month later, Scott is no longer ambulatory. I see the red Cavalier of the palliative care doctor parked on the road. Dr. Goldman is short and thin, a wisp of a man, like a spirit who blows in and out, bringing comfort and warmth. Dr. Goldman is the same age as Scott. He has a gentle voice and a warm, generous handshake. Carrie tells me that he is always available for them. "He's the lifesaver in all of this," she says.

Today Scott is holding on for dear life. I can now identify the cars that crowd the double driveway and overflow onto the street. Each day, the blue Avalon, the silver Volvo, the green minivan, and the eggplant A-8 are arranged like Dinky cars in the driveway. The passengers wear different clothes, but the ashen faces remain the same: Scott's brother and sister-in-law, who is six months pregnant; Carrie's brother; Scott's two best friends and their partners. Scott's mother, struggling with her own health, brings bouquets of red roses and white freesia, sprays of seeded eucalyptus, and alstroemeria, while Carrie's mother, herself a breast cancer survivor, spends her days and nights in the back sunroom, making herself available to cook and clean or visit with the friends who come at all hours.

I drop over to see Carrie when the parking lot is empty. She insists that she has everything she needs. No flowers, no cakes, no casseroles, no books. "The freezer is overflowing with food. Please take some," she says.

I offer to take the dog out for a walk.

"Mulligan is getting more walks than she ever did before. But thanks anyway." Carrie's voice is a monotone. I hug her and feel her diaphragm against mine, her thin ribcage heaving.

Carrie's mother is home during one of my visits. The doorbell is taped over. Mulligan is living with friends. "Scott can't take startling noises anymore," Carrie's mother tells me. "The sound of Mully's claws on the floor, the doorbell, footsteps, music, the vibrations of the floorboards — all disturb him. He does not like to be surprised. I always announce my presence before I go into his room so that he can hear me before he sees me. He is so scared of Mully jumping on his bed because of the pain."

I cover my mouth with my hand. I am shocked by what she is saying.

"Dr. Goldman is still trying to manage his pain," Carrie's mother continues, "without making him too drugged or stuporous." Her voice is heavy. I am without words.

"Carrie knows he is dying now. She feels it is her mission in life to take care of him. Carrie has been administering all his medications — the red, blue, and white tablets, the capsules, the injections. I tell her that Scott has touched a lot of people and that his short life will be remembered."

I nod in agreement. I look at the pictures of Scott on the fireplace mantel. Scott dressed in a tuxedo: blond hair, blue eyes, arm around his brother. And another of Scott in a sweatsuit, the stem of a red rose in his mouth.

• • •

In the children's bereavement groups I used to conduct at Bereaved Families of Ontario, there was a question box. Children could write anonymous questions on slips of colored paper and put them in the box. On curled pieces of yellow paper I read, "Why did my mummy have to die?" "Why did Daddy get so sick?" "Why couldn't the doctors help my sister?" The words choke me. Why indeed?

Parents are scared to tell their children about death, about illness. They do not have the answers to those questions. Children paint pictures of death — bogeymen, ghosts, creatures of the night, monsters. Death in black and white. Death lurking behind curtains, under beds, in cemeteries.

I decide to take a walk in Mount Pleasant Cemetery on a bright, sunny afternoon. I read the burial stones. I stare at a budding plant that has just been transplanted from a pot to the ground. Within its seeds is the potential for life, for renewal, for regeneration. Dead, dry leaves sweep along the pavement.

I remember Billy, a blond, blue-eyed nine-year-old whose parents were separated. He and his eleven-year-old brother were living with their mother but had regular contact with their father. Billy loved hockey, baseball, Superman comics, gummy bears, and Pokémon cards. So did his dad, he said. Billy always wore a baseball cap backwards. So did his dad, he said. Two years after his parents separated, his father was diagnosed with a virulent form of melanoma. After the diagnosis, he was treated with six months of chemotherapy.

As it became obvious that the treatment wasn't working,

Billy's father moved to the family cottage in Muskoka, a cottage area two hours north of Toronto. Billy and his brother visited him on weekends with their mother. During one of their last visits, Billy and his brother were called into their father's room. Their father told them that he was going to die shortly and he wanted them to know that he loved them dearly and always would, that they should always love their mother, that one day their mother might remarry and that they should welcome that man into their lives. He died a week later.

All of this I learned at the first session of a seven-week bereavement group. In the second session, when children were encouraged to bring in family photos and memorabilia, Billy brought in a scrapbook that contained photos and news clippings about his father, who had worked for a radio station and was also an avid mountaineer and hiker.

"This is my father when he climbed a very big mountain before my mom and dad were married. This is my mom and dad at their wedding. This is my dad dressed up at Hallowe'en — doesn't he look goofy? And this is my dad and me going to watch a baseball game." As he spoke, his voice cracked and tears began to form. Julie, a ten-year-old sitting beside him, handed Billy a tissue.

In a session on funerals, Billy described the church full of hundreds of people. In his picture he drew a bunch of circles and called it "a parade of crying men and women." In the sky, he made "angry clouds with angry faces."

As the sessions progressed, Billy opened up more about his inner feelings. He said he hated the changes in his life, he hated his mother's new boyfriend, and he even hated his mother sometimes. He was mad at his father for dying and leaving him in the hands of his mother and this other man. In his family drawing, splotches of thick black paint covered everyone except the family dog.

For Billy, a year after his father's death, life was still an emotional roller coaster. His behavior at home and school was punctuated by outbursts, temper tantrums, and defiance. In the group he talked about his moodiness and his inability to "be good." At the final session, he said he loved meeting other kids whose mothers or fathers had died, because it made him feel that he wasn't "bad" or "evil" for having all those weird ideas and feelings. "I feel more normal now and I can at least tell my mom when I get mad at her," he wrote on his evaluation.

When the group ended, Billy saw a therapist individually for a few months. The last I heard, he was doing well at both home and school.

• • •

Freud said that in the unconscious, everyone is convinced of his or her own immortality. I would say that not only is our own death inconceivable, but so too are the deaths of those we love.

Loss is a terror. Loss reverberates with fears of abandonment. Death reminds us of our own mortality. It is a topic to avoid. The unconscious is pleased to cooperate in our denial.

Yet loss is part of life, and the pain of grief is as much a part of relationships as the ecstasy of love. It is the price we pay for the intimacy we have with others. Grieving is the process of converting the presence of a significant other into an absence, of transforming actuality into memory. It is the task of each bereaved person to construct a framework of memories, a framework that will endure over time and space.

Reality demands that we gradually withdraw our psychic energy from a loved one who has died. Yet none of us willingly gives up this attachment. Instead we try to turn away or deny reality, clinging desperately to the lost person. Eventually we are forced to disengage, albeit in a rather piecemeal manner, and life resumes its zigzag course.

Bereaved children grieve differently from their parents. Their reactions are less verbal, less well-defined. Lacking in sophisticated cognitive skills and intellectual maturity, their responses are frequently expressed in a (dis)array of behaviors or in play. They refuse to eat, have temper tantrums, refuse to go to school, withdraw into themselves. They approach and withdraw, unable to sustain the emotional intensity of adults.

I remember attending the funeral of a friend whose husband had died. When her ten-year-old daughter looked at her watch and asked to go play with her friends, "since school will be out now," her mother was mortified. I reminded her that after forty-eight hours of tears and emotion, after strangers shaking her hand and saying "I'm sorry," after two days of visitation *and* the funeral *and* now the reception, maybe this was all her daughter could handle for the time being. It was not a question of disrespect.

In an environment of silence, created by adults who withhold information in the guise of protection, children manufacture their own ideas and explanations in order to once again create order out of disorder. Lacking a philosophical or theological framework in which to place their ideas, their fantasies and musings are often more frightening than the facts their parents know. Children need to be reassured that they did not cause the death, that there will be a minimum of disruption to their lives, that the dead will not seek revenge at night, and that they will continue to be loved and taken care of by the surviving parent.

• • •

I first met the Reverend Timothy Elliott when we both sat in meetings to determine Wellspring's policies and procedures. Later, when I became program director, I asked Tim to facilitate a series, the Spiritual Dimensions of Cancer. In the B. B. Bargoon room on the second floor, Tim's six-foot frame was crunched into a low loveseat, his knees almost tickling his chest, but his ear was attuned to the pain of six men and women discussing questions of faith, fear, and dying.

Today I am meeting Tim for lunch at the Waterside Sports Club, where Tim is a member. As I look out over the chilly waters of Lake Ontario from inside the dining room, seagulls perform acrobatic feats in their play for survival. The clouds are low, gray-capped, as if to warn of freezing rain or snow.

I am lost in visions of our cottage on Lake Temagami as Tim approaches. "Hello, how nice to see you again," he says, extending his arm in a welcoming handshake. "How long has it been? Two, three years?"

Tim is dressed in a dark suit with a burgundy-striped tie. His graying hair is still damp from the shower after his game of tennis. I notice more salt than pepper in his beard. His voice relaxes me as I wait for him to adjust his body into the chair.

We have much catching up to do: my practice, my ongoing

involvement at Wellspring, the Out of the Cold program at his church, preparations for the Christmas season, the politics of charitable boards, family affairs. As we reminisce about colleagues from Wellspring, I study Tim surreptitiously. I respect him; he is a man with the insight of a trained psychotherapist, the compassion of a minister, and the wisdom of a sage.

The plates of food arrive, and we indulge for a few moments in the silent pleasures of eating.

"I see you haven't been fed in a while," Tim says, noticing my greasy fingers.

"Sure tastes good when you're hungry," I reply. "I just came back from a workout myself." I am restraining myself in other ways, sitting on a question, pacing out the meal until it can be asked.

"I have a question for you," I finally say.

"Go ahead, whatever it is," he volunteers.

I launch into a description of Scott's illness and his three-month struggle with cancer. But I cannot complete my sentences, staring at the tomatoes and red peppers swimming in a pool of oil in front of me.

"So what's the question?" Tim asks innocently.

"How do you deal with this? This one won't go away, Tim. I found myself getting so *angry*. I've just been thinking it's not fair. It's not fair that someone so young, so vital, so full of potential should die. It's awful when an older person dies, but it's horrific when it's someone who has so much to give. How do you make sense of this?"

Tim does not respond immediately. I look up for a second and his eyes meet mine. "Mavis, there are many systems of religious, philosophical, and theosophical thought that all grapple with the question of life and death. And we all struggle ourselves with the need to make sense of pain and suffering. We also know that there are certain people who attain a degree of acceptance and peace in their final days, and others who do not. But no matter what our philosophical or religious faith, no matter to what extent we acept death as a reality, we can't deny ourselves the range of emotions that accompany loss — sadness, rage, pain, loneliness."

He pauses and then continues, "You know death is all around us all the time, and some of us who do this kind of work have our antennae tuned in to that frequency more than others. If you work at a place like Wellspring, then you automatically open yourself up."

I look outside and the sun is burning through the clouds. From my vantage point by the window, I catch a glimpse of something silver floating in the water by the dock. A dead fish. A seagull pokes at its head. I look away.

"Mavis, there are days when I feel that it doesn't make sense and there is no point trying to make sense of it. Death *is* a tradegy. It *is* awful and it *isn't* fair. Sometimes it is important to rage at the injustice of a life cut short. I too sometimes rage for what I perceive as unjust."

Tim proceeds to tell me about a late winter afternoon when he and a friend were walking along the boardwalk in the Beach neighborhood. As the coughing water billowed against the rocks, he began to shout obscenities. "You know how good that felt? To be able to let it out, let it go? Of course, my friend thought that I had lost it, but for me it was an important ritual."

I smile at Tim, trying to imagine this respectful, and mild-mannered man in his ministerial garb cursing at the unforgiving waters of Lake Ontario.

"You must know when it gets too much and you must take care of yourself. There are always those who touch us more. I cope by becoming clinically detached. And that too passes."

We continue to discuss the challenges of this work. Then Tim says he must leave and we pay the bill. We hug briefly before parting and he disappears into his car.

The sun is bright on the waters. I decide to walk along the dock. I think about Tim's words. *It's okay to rage. It is unjust.* A mallard and her young brood coast along the shoreline, nearly camouflaged by debris.

I remember the bereavement workshop for professionals that Anne and I gave at Wellspring, about the need to create meaning through rituals, the importance of journal-writing, artwork, and spiritual beliefs in helping turn events of loss into something positive. We discussed alternative mourning rituals that some of us had tried in our groups. Sue mentioned a ritual service her group had conducted after a member died. I described the candle-lighting ceremony and the moment of silence that I had incorporated into my groups. Lorna talked about a journal of memorial services. We all agreed that it was important for us to talk about our own, personal losses, so Anne led us through an activity on this subject — a personal grief timeline. At the end of the evening, we all reaffirmed the belief that healing does occur in time, and that we could not spare our members this critical psychological process.

I know the words. I rehearse them in front of the mirror. I

repeat them to myself in the car. But sometimes they lose their power and I am overwhelmed by the magnitude of death.

The day after my lunch with Tim, Lawlor and I attend Scott's funeral. The church is packed with people, old and young, men and women. The minister's white hair glows from the pulpit as the family walks down the aisle: Scott's mother and father; Scott's brother and sister-in-law; Carrie's father, mother, and brother; Carrie and Mulligan. When the minister speaks, there is only the sound of sniffling and nose-blowing.

"Tears are an appreciation of love at the loved one's death. Tears are okay. But let us not only cry, for this is also a celebration of life. Yes, a life too short, but nevertheless a life that was full in its thirty-two years. It was Scott's wish that his family and friends celebrate, through laughter and tears, his life and his memories."

• • •

Another cruel blow. Eighteen months after his recovery from a cerebral aneurysm, my friend Ninna had noticed a lump on Sid's head. The doctors were afraid to remove the lump under general anesthesia; it was too soon after his aneurysm, so they used a local anesthetic.

Two months later, as Ninna tells me during our market expedition, the wound is seeping, oozing; the scar is not healing.

This time they will give him a general anesthetic. Ninna and Mikala, Sid and Ninna's daughter, are given tranquilizers the night before the surgery. Friends leave messages on their voice mail. We all await the outcome nervously. An alphabetical call-back system has been organized. All I can think about is that Sid and Ninna are my oldest friends in Toronto, like family. It was through them that I met Lawlor.

The surgery is successful. Sid has come out of the anesthesia without any apparent disability. He can recite his name, address, and telephone number; he knows that he is at St. Michael's Hospital; he can repeat seven digits forward and backward; he can move his fingers and toes, cough, and count to twenty.

Three months later, the lump has returned. Sid is diagnosed with a sarcoma.

"This is an aggressive bastard," the doctor says.

The plastic surgeon refers Sid to an oncologist, who looks over the three-inch-thick dossier. "This man has been through a lot. I'm afraid we might have to try chemotherapy, but I will have to speak to his neurologist about his general health."

A team of specialists gathers in the conference room at the end of the corridor. The door remains closed for several hours.

Ninna calls a family meeting to discuss the options. A feud erupts between Ninna and Sid's estranged brother and sister, Josh and Hazel. They accuse her of trying to kill Sid by denying him chemotherapy. Ninna is too tired, drained. Two and a half years of hospital visits, sleepless nights, and anxiety has weakened her defenses.

Josh demands to speak to the doctor — any doctor, he does not care. Ninna gives up the battle; she is too exhausted to fight. The oncologist is noncommittal; liability is his concern. Finally Josh backs down when he sees how fragile his brother's tormented body is.

Over the next four months, Sid loses weight, loses lucidity, and loses his will to live. Tumors erupt on his neck, his legs, his collarbone. His body is ravaged with disease.

Sid begins to refuse food. I make homemade soups for him. I want to nourish him back to health. I puree broccoli, carrots, squash, potatoes, cauliflower, and deliver Tupperware containers of wholesome broth twice a week. "Sid loves your soup," Ninna says, but he is eating only half a cup a day.

Sid's robust frame is dwindling. He looks dwarfed by the queen-size bed with its cobalt blue and sunny yellow duvet cover from Denmark. For moments his mind becomes crystal clear, uncluttered, and then he relapses, retreating into a darkness of silence, moving only his eyes and squeezing a hand in recognition.

"Sid, you've got to try harder to eat," everyone is pleading. Anger bubbles up. Sid is not fighting hard enough.

Ninna plans a birthday party for Sid. This is the first time he has agreed to a party for his birthday. All his friends will come and celebrate his fifty-five years of life.

Fifty-five friends and relatives attend the party. There are no gifts. Lawlor brings Sid an eagle feather he found on Vancouver Island, bound with a red-and-white string from a meditation retreat. He has attached to it a letter for Sid and Ninna.

Platters of food arrive. People mill around the dining-room table that holds black bread and *gravad laks*, bagels and cream cheese, curried herring and *rodbede salat*. Aquavit with beer chasers. *Kransekage*. A Danish–Jewish celebration, another annual event.

Ben, a physician and close friend of twenty-five years, comes down the stairs, his underarms soaked in perspiration. "I don't think Sid is going to last another twenty-four hours," he says. Everyone speaks in whispers.

What does a dying person look like? I am scared to ascend the stairs. What haunting image will I see? I have never been this close to death. I want to see Sid, to wish him a happy birthday, to say goodbye.

I count the stairs as I climb. One, two, three . . . twelve, thirteen, fourteen. The room is cool in spite of the outdoor heat. Maple leaves rustle against the window, from which I can see the murky waters of Lake Ontario. I remember the day Sid and Ninna purchased this house. "We've bought a house," Sid said to his friends. "We're Beachers now. No more downtown living."

On the dresser beside the bed sit three miniature elephants — an ivory one with elongated tusks, an ebony one trumpeting with its trunk in the air, and a striped one of an African wood. There are also a picture of Sid, Ninna, and Mikala from Christmas 1990 and a half-drunk glass of water with a bendable straw. On the walls, messages from Ninna: "Sidney, you are at home." "Your water is behind the tray." "Check your watch for the time." On the desk beside the dresser is a book of messages from Ninna to the homecare nurse; from the homemaker to Ninna; from Heather and Ian to Ninna; from Ninna to Julia, the Interlink worker.

Sid's eyelids flutter and I am not sure if he is awake. I watch his chest rise and fall in measured breaths. I clasp his thin fingers in mine. His hand is warm and weightless. He opens his eyes.

"It's Mavis, Sid," I say, leaning over to kiss his forehead. "There are lots of people downstairs. They have all come to wish you happy birthday. You have many, many friends, you and

Ninna." I am talking in baby syllables as though Sid can no longer digest complex sandwiches of sentences. He smiles. I sense rather than feel a gentle squeeze in my palm.

"Is it all right to sit on the bed, Sid?" I ask and gently lower myself onto the mattress. Sid's breathing is shallow. He pulls his hand out of mine and extends his arm into the air. He is looking at his fingers as if decoding a telegraphic signal. His fingers form silhouettes against the wall — a rabbit, a cat, a dog.

Sid, where are you? I wonder. He no longer responds to my voice. He is searching for something in the motion of his fingers.

Sid, are you at peace? Are you in pain? Are you aware of what is happening around you? Every time he closes his eyes, I fear he will not open them again.

"Maybe you are tired, Sid," I say out loud. "So many people, so many handshakes; so many smells, perfumes, sounds of foot-steps; so much pressure on the bed, on your tired being. Too much for you, Sid. I will leave you in peace." I lean over and kiss his forehead.

I pull back and take one more look at Sid. I know it will be my last. I inhale deeply. He lies in peaceful repose.

Sid died thirty-four hours later, just past midnight. Ninna was lying beside him on the bed. His breathing simply stopped. There was no fanfare, no fireworks. A quiet passing away. Within forty-eight hours, the same group of friends assembled at the hall of A Simple Alternative for the funeral service. A rabbi recited the prayer for the dead — the same rabbi who as hospi-tal chaplain had visited Sid after his aneurysm. We followed in a single line, like schoolchildren, to the cemetery. It was a hot, muggy day in a summer of hot, muggy days. There was no respite from the heat. We entered a new section of the cemetery that lacked the shade of mature trees.

"I picked a spot near the flowering shrubs. I know Sid would be happy with that," Ninna said, standing by the table after the service. "That was a nice service, wasn't it?"

Passed away, I kept thinking. *He just passed away*. The words went through my head, over and over again. He closed his eyes and passed on — on to another plane, another, invisible sphere. In peace, he simply passed on.

In my journal I compose a poem entitled "Death."

Death has no respect,
no respect for the crying infants, the young, the needy.
A final blow and the last breath is chopped off. Final,
no second chance.

Death has no respect
for the weather.
The people gather in flurries
blown across the parking lot, the snow swirls
Yet inside the church the season is eternal
The choirboys in their frilly collars swelling with
upturned faces
except for the mischievous one who wrinkles his nose
perplexed
at the crowds who fill the pews.

The sniveling, the frail, the aged,
couples in their Sunday best
paying respects to disrespectful
death.
The whispered voices, the muffled sighs,
the crowd sweeps together
briefly and disperse,
forgetting the names, the flames, the pains
of the family
who stand behind, waiting for the storm to end.

• • •

The graduate metastatic group decides to have a retreat. They wish to discuss death. They want to talk about dying, about wills, living wills, and power of attorney. They want to plan funeral arrangements and memorial services. They are still fighting for control.

Days prior to the retreat, I call a colleague who works for Interlink Community Care Nurses, a service provider for cancer patients. "Brenda, tell me about palliative work. I need some assistance here."

I have never met Brenda face to face, but we have had several phone conversations about mutual cases. Her voice is soft and subdued as she speaks. She poses a number of questions for the group to think about: In the parting of life, what are the things that can be done to create a history of family memories or to compensate for past regrets? What needs to be said and done so that there is no unfinished family business? What can be said and done to ensure a sense of family continuity?

"It doesn't have to be just a death sentence waiting to happen," she says. "I think of it as a gift from the dying person to their family. There is valuable time left to develop future possibilities through the creation of a shared past." Then Brenda goes on to describe the death of her mother and how her last few days provided precious time for the family together.

In the peaceful surroundings of Edwards Gardens, the group assembles for the day. We ease into our chairs and I lead them through a guided visualization. Then we do a few exercises. I have them work through the task of the "treasure box," which forces them to think about the most important items they would choose if they were stranded on an island. Quietly they write and draw their responses before sharing them in the group.

Later we approach the work of the day and the discussion begins.

Carole: "It is not death that worries me. It's the pain."

Tove: "For me, it is about dying alone, not being surrounded by a circle of friends or family."

Terry: "For me, it is about leaving this world with dignity. Not being seen as weak and fragile, incontinent, and all that awful stuff. I want to be remembered as I was in my life, not in my final days."

Sarah: "I agree. And then there's the whole issue of dying at home. What is best for the children? To see you sick at the end?"

Terry: "For me, that's the ultimate question. I really prefer to die at home, but I need to be reassured that my family is really all right with that. And then I still think, will my husband really want to sleep in the room in which I died? Will they remember me by those images?"

Carole: "But how do you remember your parents and your grandparents? Do you only visualize them at the end, sick and dying? I certainly don't."

Tove: "Of course, your children will want you at home. It is easier for them, it makes living more 'normal.'"

Sarah: "Perhaps we don't give our families enough credit. My kids are already eighteen and twenty. When I really think about it, I'm sure they can manage it."

Terry: "But what about the pain? I need to know that my family will be supported by a team if I choose to be at home. I don't want to put them in an awkward or unprotected position."

Tove: "You're right, Terry. Aside from the psychological stuff, there's the practical side of pain management, medications, and on and on."

My mind drifts . . .

My father's death was quick — no goodbyes, no farewells. My grandmother's death was slow and lingering. My mother grew old as she watched her mother die. I still see my grandmother as a thin envelope of flesh, even though throughout her life her body was round and powerful.

Dignity. The wish to be remembered as one lived. The last illusion of control versus the final surrender. The ultimate control of one's destiny: to choose one's death. Dignity. To die with aplomb, with style, with panache? To die in peace? With friends and family? Alone?

The women on this retreat are posing essential questions and wrestling with profound issues. They know they are unable to choose *when* they die, but they want to have choices about *where* and *how* they die. At home with palliative support? In a hospital? In a community hospice center? They want to decide for themselves before they bring their ideas home to their families. It is often fear of the family's response that prevents open and honest dialogue about such important decisions.

If a person chooses to die at home, for example, it is critical that family members be involved so that they can be fully informed about pain management, disease progression, medications, and the practical details of everyday functioning. Without this support and collaboration, there is fear, resentment, and family stress. It is also important that family members be taught what to expect psychologically, both for the dying person and for their loved ones: a whirlwind of emotions rather than neatly defined stages and phases.

For the dying person, there are also choices about one's legacy, one's link in the intergenerational family chain. I recall my conversation with Brenda. *In parting from life, what things can be done to create a history of family memories or to compensate for past regrets? What needs to be said and done so that there is no unfinished business? What can be said and done to ensure a sense of family continuity? Dying can be thought of as a progression rather than an end. Think of "moving towards" rather than a "final parting."*

At the end of the day, Terry says laughingly, "I've got it! There's this nice woman who comes into my husband's shop. The kids know her because they've met her several times at the store, and they think she's kind of cool. So maybe I can arrange for her to take my place when I'm gone."

"Now that you mention it," Carole adds, "I was thinking my

widowed cousin would make a great mother for my kids, because she already has a relationship with them. Maybe I should set her up as my fill-in, like write it into the will or something."

• • •

I am sitting in a large auditorium in my second year at McGill University. Professor Ron Melzack is talking about pain. To the sea of faces shaded in darkness, he says confidently, "Pain is more than nerve endings. Look at the phenomenon of the phantom limb. There is no limb, yet there is pain. Look at the results of studies on the impact of placebo medication. There is always a psychological component to pain."

Is this true of cancer pain? Can it be prevented by psychological measures alone? The answer is no.

Pain saps strength, drains the life force, bruises our sense of self-worth. Pain deprives one of sleep and appetite. Unrelieved, prolonged pain tilts one toward the direction of permanent sleep.

I have spoken to physicians who tell me that unrelieved pain is the result of improper pain medication. "Why?" I ask earnestly. "Why do patients continue to suffer? I hear it all the time. And it is cancer patients' biggest fear."

I am told that the patient is scared of losing control. The patient is scared of side effects. The patient is afraid to maintain the prescribed dosage.

"And what about the physicians?" I ask. "What is the problem there?"

I am told that the physician is not always well informed about current trends. The physician is reluctant to prescribe the necessary dosage because of the opiate substrate.

I tell the members in the metastatic group, "You have choices around sedation. You are entitled to adequate pain management. You can insist on marijuana, morphine, or whatever cocktail of drugs it takes to relieve your pain."

I have learned through my work that most people are not afraid of dying. What most people fear is dying in pain. While there have been considerable advances in palliative care and pain management, there continue to be ignorance and myth about how to titrate, monitor, and adjust dosages of complex pain medication. Doctors who do not specialize in this field are still reluctant to prescribe the dosage necessary to alleviate pain or are not well enough informed about the combinations of pain inhibitors in use today.

On the other hand, patients and family members are also reluctant about administering the recommended dosage, out of fear of losing lucidity in the final days or becoming so drug-dulled by the medication that they cannot interact with their loved ones.

It is clearly a complicated process to balance and manage pain. Psychological factors such as fear and stress are also known to contribute to the body's response to pain. Distressed family members and caretakers can have a direct impact on a patient's pain levels, either exacerbating or alleviating the body's responses. Therefore it is important to persist in requesting relief from specialists and to establish trusting relationships with caregivers and health professionals.

• • •

I have decided to put together a family album, a scrapbook of my family legacy. I am anticipating the need to create some meaning in my personal life. I replay what was discussed on the retreat. Am I rushing the process?

I fly to Montreal to spend a weekend with my mother. I feel a sense of desperation, of time running out. I must record the names, draw a family tree before there is no time. Whose time? Mine? My mother's? I have already lost the account of my father's family; there are no family historians left. My mother is an only child. There are no aunts, uncles, or cousins to confirm the stories.

I look at a photo of my mother in her wedding dress. I see a radiant young woman. And then I pull out another one of her at my graduation, where I am the age she was at the time of her marriage and she is the age I am today. The passage of time recorded in images. "We have made it at least this far," I hear myself saying.

9

I stop in at WonderWorks on Harbord Street to buy some Japanese incense for Lawlor. A cornucopia of New Age products delights the eye: lunar wall calendars, goddess knowledge cards, silver and pewter pendants, rainbow crystals, Willow Moon batik T-shirts, temporary tattoos, chimes, handmade soaps and creams, oils and essences, miniature sculptures, and CDs and tapes celebrating goddesses, crones, healers, and the healed. The shelves are stacked with books on the occult, on Jewish spiritualism, on meditation practices, on Christian mysticism. I notice a slim volume on Jewish rituals and flip through the pages of familiar traditional blessings alternating with contemporary revisions and additions.

The woman behind the cash has a round face with clear blue

eyes, a clear complexion, and no makeup. Her black dance slippers beneath balloon trousers remind me of a Chinese doll. She introduces herself as Lillian and asks if she can help me in any way while I browse. She does not recognize me and wonders if this is the first time I have been to the store.

I ask her about Japanese incense, but she informs me that they stock only Chinese incense and sticks made in New Mexico, with names like Sierra Cedar, Egyptian Musk, Enchanted Forest, Sandalwood, Lotus Moon, and Lavender Fields. I tell her my husband is very particular, so I'll just continue to look around.

My eye is attracted by an indoor water fountain made of black slate and wood. Someone has placed a few stones and a miniature moose on the slate top. The water flows over a Chinese flower-holder containing a sprig of yellow freesia and a white tea rose. Haiku water ballet. Lillian is excited by my interest in the Water Muse fountain. "It is very Zen, the nicest fountain we've seen around. It can be set up anywhere in five minutes and requires no special plumbing."

I think the fountain will be inspirational for my writing and decide to buy the smaller version. Then I study the bookshelves in closer detail and leaf through some of the titles. One in particular catches my attention: *Kaddish*, by Leon Weiseltier, a hardcover volume with a white paper jacket, that fits into my hand as comfortably as a prayer book. I read the fly-leaf of the dust cover: "When Leon Weiseltier's father died, he began to say the daily Kaddish, mourner's prayer, for 365 days. This book is his journey and dedication."

I walk to the counter and Lillian takes the items from me one by one: a jar of lavender Blue Corn cleansing grains, the fountain, and three books: *Handwriting*, Michael Ondaatje's latest collection of poems, *Kaddish*, and a book on parenting by Jon Kabat-Zinn and his wife.

"Interesting choice," Lillian comments, as she rings in the book by the Kabat-Zinns. "It's a different take on parenting compared to the usual stuff." She leans forward across the counter, and I catch a whiff of patchouli from her sweater.

"I was thinking this might be a good gift for a friend's daughter," I say, ensuring that she does not think I am buying it for myself.

Lillian carefully wraps the items and puts them in two large paper shopping bags. "Be careful with the handles," she warns me.

As I am about to leave, my eye lights on a table of stones. After reading the descriptions, I choose four of them: moonstone, malachite, amethyst, and chrysoprase. I am protected now. I carefully select an emerald-green silk pouch with a tie-dyed flower on it to guard my stones.

• • •

Carole begins the group today. She clasps her belly and says that she senses a recurrence of her cancer — again, the sixth time in fifteen years. "I am tired of fighting. I'm no longer sure I want another round of chemo. I have done the visualization, the psychotherapy, the macrobiotic diet. I am not scared of death anymore. But I am scared of the pain of recurrence and the pain of death."

Preeya: "I am also having a hard week. I'm not yet sure if it is a cold or a reaction to the chemo, but everything aches."

Tove: "Somehow I think you have to be positive. For me, it is a question of what I can do to heal my body. I refuse to let my treatment be dictated solely by the doctors. Besides, in my case, they threw up their hands. So I went on my own search and ended up with the ozone therapy and chelation. It's what I do for myself . . ."

Carole: "Somehow I feel the group is always focusing on the positive. I came here so that I could have a place to discuss what I can't discuss with my family and friends, and what we keep avoiding here — and that's the topic of death."

Tove: "Look, I know that there is a big reality of death with metastatic disease — I'm not stupid. But I refuse to be a statistic. Statistics say that three percent survive. Well, I can be one of those three percent. I'm prepared to do anything that will increase my chances of survival. And I also believe in the power of nature and diet and the force of will."

Lily: "I understand both of you, Carole and Tove. Carole, you say you are tired and fatigued and maybe even fed up with the struggle. Yet you have been battling for fifteen years. You are a role model for me. Of course you're ambivalent. Of course you're tired. So am I. I have sharp pains in my chest and a reaction to this Cook's catheter. I can't get in touch with my oncologist. I'm frustrated by all of it. Yet I feel 'out of the wilderness' in terms of my body. Now I'm working on my life force. I *want* to live. So I'm doing some things to heal myself spiritually. I've done the chemo and the diet for my physician; now I'm doing something for me."

A week later, Carole discusses a new book she has read, *A Cancer Battle Plan*. She has arranged to see a Chinese doctor who is also a herbalist, as well as a second physician, who practices Tibetan herbal medicine. Preeya is doing reading on healing prayers. Tove is pursuing her spiritual exercises. Lily is still convinced that the "miracle" cases may no longer be the exceptions.

My mother calls to inquire if I have read a new book called *Cancer Prevention and Diet*. "It says that grilling and barbecuing food is unhealthy. You know your sister and Peter, they love their barbecued chicken. Maybe that is what caused your sister's cancer," she suggests.

I roll my eyes in the privacy of my blue-and-yellow kitchen. My mother hears my silence. "It says you should boil potatoes instead . . ."

"Mom, it's okay."

"I think you should read it, sweetheart. It doesn't hurt. I'll send you a copy."

"Thanks, Mom."

A week later my mother calls to tell me she has seen Barbara. "Barbara Koffman. You know, Sonny and Gail's daughter. She lives in London, England, now and she's visiting."

My memories of Barbara Koffman roll across the screen of my mind. A chubby girl in a turquoise snowsuit with a yellow toque, red cheeks, and a missing front tooth.

"She's studying kinesiology," my mother continues. "She came over for coffee with Gail yesterday. I served that wonderful coffeecake recipe you gave me, the one with the pecan streusel topping. Delicious. Anyway, Barbara was explaining to me how it's not good to wear electronic watches and that the old manual wind-ups are much healthier. It has to do with balancing your body. Now which watch are you wearing these days, dear? Maybe you should think about this."

"Yes, Mother."

• • •

Thirty years ago, when I was listening to the Beatles, the Rolling Stones, and the Doors, experimenting with marijuana and burning incense in the basement of my parents' house, a woman on the west coast of the United States was trying to understand the healing powers of the mind. Catherine Ponder, a minister of the nondenominational Unity faith, was not spending her time reading Leonard Cohen, Joseph Heller, or Germaine Greer. Instead she was writing books on prosperity and healing.

According to Ponder, "There is a divine current within you that carries healing power." All one needs to do is tap into the conscious, subconscious, and superconscious minds through prayer, affirmation, and spiritual study, and the process of bodily healing will begin. In a book entitled *The Healing Secrets of the Ages*, Ponder writes,

> These secret teachings have to do with 12 mind powers located within the vital nerve centers in your body, which greatly affect your health, either constructively or destructively, depending upon how you are using these mind powers. . . . The number 12 has always been regarded as a sacred number of completion in the development of man's higher powers.

And further,

> References to the 12 mind powers in man are found in the oldest documents dealing with human beliefs and practices. The ancient Greeks, Persians, Egyptians and Hindus felt that every part of the body had a secret meaning, and their priests placed statues of man's body in their temples in order to study its secret meaning.

I lie in bed reading Ponder on the healing powers of judgment, love, imaging, understanding, elimination, and will. I become a patchwork of disconnected squares. I read that every movement, every act, contains a potential for negative impact on my body. Even my speech can determine my fate.

> The body feeds on man's words. When those words are life-giving, they are health-producing. . . . When words are spoken that describe disease as a reality, those words unconsciously set in motion disintegrating forces in the body which shatter the strongest organism if they are not counteracted by constructive words.

I dream about causing a patient of mine ill-harm and undue suffering — that I am responsible for throat and chest diseases because of my reckless flinging about of words; that I have irritated nasal passages by speaking in a rasping, angry voice; that I have caused shriveling of cells, hardening of arteries, and congestion of the flow of life-fluids with thoughts of bitterness and condemnation. I am doomed by my actions to die. I pray for salvation and that my words, tossed like refuse into a garbage can, will go unheeded. My days are numbered by my misdeeds.

In the group the next morning, Lily tells me that she is enchanted with Ponder and invites the other members to read her books. "She is such an inspiration to me. I want to focus my energy on what I *can* do to heal myself. Ponder gives me some concrete exercises I can do myself."

She elaborates on the similarities between Catherine Ponder and Caroline Myss, a contemporary writer who shares similar views about the development of human consciousness and spirituality. Myss portrays herself as a medical intuitive who describes for people their physical diseases as well as the energy dysfunctions within their bodies. She uses "energy medicine" to treat the body and spirit. Like Ponder, she also examines the potential for transformation through attitudes about healing.

While Myss is not herself a healer, she writes about "the energy field that permeates and surrounds the body, picks up information about dramatic childhood events, behavior patterns, even superstitious beliefs," all of which she believes have a bearing on a person's healing. In her book *Why People Don't Heal and How They Can*, she offers a number of recommendations for self-cure, beginning with a personal understanding of how one's body and life reflect the energy of the chakras, *sefirot*, or sacraments. She suggests spiritual practices in addition to a healthy lifestyle for integrating mind and body healing, for example, learning to say no, setting realistic goals, developing willpower, cultivating grace, and visualizing your chakras.

Do our bodies become our biographies, as Myss states? If a

woman's body is the first environment of life, does it follow that we pass our genetic inheritance of sickness to our children in a one-to-one correspondence? And if we contaminate our environment, do we necessarily contaminate our bodies?

Some people believe that we are in a symbiotic relationship with the earth. We need plants and trees for oxygen, their byproduct. Plants and trees need man for carbon dioxide, our byproduct. What man considers negative is positive for the earth, and vice versa.

Some people believe that the sacred places of the earth's landscape, or energy fields, mirror the positions of the body's landscape as measured by our chakras, or energy centers. Some people believe that if we live only in the upper half of our body, using only the higher chakras, then we deprive the earth of what it needs — the grounding of interaction.

• • •

During a time of vulnerability, when we are faced with serious illness and the prospect of our own mortality, when the trauma of what Lacan calls the Real (that which lies outside of language and resists symbolization) is inescapable, we are pushed into corners from which we cannot escape. It is at these points of juncture, of trauma and crisis, that we are more receptive to new ideas. It is at these times that our minds curl and stretch around alternative views, growing in directions that we would otherwise ignore, or even deride.

Preeya, Susan, Tove, Lily, and the others all complain about being bombarded by magazines and books from well-intentioned relatives and friends expounding the positive outcomes of shark cartilage, polarity therapy, various herbs and diets, and energy life therapies, among others. I go into the health food store for some groceries and I read about CoQ-10, a new immune-system booster. I walk into bookstores in Kathmandu, in Santa Fe, in Tel Aviv, and I read about new cures for cancer treatment. In 1994, the Ontario Breast Cancer Exchange Project published *A Guide to Unconventional Cancer Therapies*, which documented all the available alternative treatments being used.

Some people search out New Age rhetoric to guide their journeys, feeling fortified by a belief in the power of these promises, while others suffer tremendous guilt because they feel unable to convert to this new wave of therapies. How do we make sense of this? How can we analyze the radical transformation of people whose previous lives were, for the most part, conventional and mainstream, who now meditate every day, follow vegetarian or macrobiotic diets, or travel to clinics in other countries in search of non-toxic cancer regimes? Is it simply a refusal to accept the finality of a poor prognosis or is it belief in a miracle cure? Is it a need to assert or regain some sense of control in the face of an uncontrollable cellular destiny?

My colleagues and friends tell me that many motives are possible: an attempt to regain a sense of self-management in reaction to perceived lack of control, the need to take an active part in one's treatment regimen, the addition of therapeutic activities to counterbalance a physically persistent disease.

"What does it matter?" demands Lydia. "If it gives people a sense of hope and control over their disease, what does it matter?"

"But what about all the charlatans out there? What about the cost of trips to Mexico, Switzerland, Ireland? What about the false hopes, the drained dreams and pocketbooks, the lack of ethics?" Danny asks.

"People make choices. They are free to choose. Maybe some people want a non-toxic chemo so they can have a quality of life that is not possible with conventional chemotherapy," Lydia retorts.

"Or maybe it is a refusal to accept the finality of a poor prognosis. Maybe, deep down, we never give up believing in miracles," I add.

I think of the people in my groups and wonder if it may be lack of faith in a traditional system that refuses to take a holistic approach to health and offers nothing when there are no further medical options.

Lydia brings me out of my thoughts. "I think it is also a radical statement about the mind–body connection, which is insistent, demanding attention. It says to people, 'You have to be an active participant in your treatment process.'"

Slinking into the role of devil's advocate, I say, "And what about the guilt? 'You didn't try hard enough.' 'You obviously didn't want to heal yourself.' Some of that language makes me sick."

Once again, we circle around the dilemmas of the twenty-first century: more technology, more information — and more questions.

I too struggle with my beliefs. In the workshops with Anne at Wellspring, we train cancer patients to become volunteer peer-support counselors. We insist on plurality of thinking, the importance of withholding our personal beliefs and allowing others to find their own paths.

I am trained to be silent, to listen, to suspend judgment, to censor my ideas and beliefs. My neutrality has become a second skin inside which I devote my attention to the text of speech. Yet in my work with cancer patients, I feel strained, constrained, and drained. I rattle around within walls, feeling pushed, pulled, confronted, challenged.

Lydia says, "Jung was right. The second half of one's life is devoted to a spiritual quest."

Lawlor laughs, "You go to Wellspring and you talk about meditation, visualization, and the mind–body connection, and you're convincing. They don't know about your skepticism." Lawlor is a true believer. He has spent most of his adult life committed to the spiritual practice of Zen Buddhism. For him, meditation is not only for the ill; it is a way of life for everyone — not a bid for health, not a barter for time. His devotion inspires me to try again.

But instead I load my bookcase with more texts on Lacan and the École Freudienne. I take workshops on German existentialism and phenomenology. I study the languages of desire, ego, and narcissism, the registers of the symbolic, the imaginary, and the real. I unravel Borromean knots and bind together death and the pleasure principle. I try to integrate the words on the pages with the experiences of Lily and Preeya, Terry and Susan.

George Papadopoulous teaches stretch classes at the fitness club where I go to strengthen and tighten my body. George has long jet hair that he ties back in a ponytail. His cheeks are dark with shadow by seven in the evening, when twelve of us gather to increase our flexibility and agility.

George is lean and muscular. His muscles bulge under his T-shirt and black shorts. He once told me that although he is Greek, he prefers to be thought of as Canadian. I looked at him quizzically when he said that.

"You know. People have queer ideas about Greek men," he laughed.

George is an excellent instructor. He can hold balance positions for several minutes and he can stretch his body in all directions. At the beginning of the class, he puts on an Andreas Vollenweider tape, and we start with a warm-up to increase blood circulation and ease the muscles into flexibility.

George says you must close your eyes and visualize the positions you are trying to achieve. He tells us that he has taught himself to walk on burning coals. He believes we can all learn to do this, if we put our minds to it. "If you truly can picture it, then you will succeed in making it happen to your body — with practice, with patience, with vision," he intones.

I sit with my legs spread apart and lean over, back straight, trying to touch the floor with my nose. I imagine my body smooth against the floor. I keep my eyes closed. For a moment I am convinced that I am a famous dancer.

George has been studying with an Indian guru for several months and is planning to go to an ashram in northern India for a year. His mantra is "stretch your body, stretch your mind."

"There must be something wrong with me," I say to Lydia. "I read *Womanspirit Rising*, *The Feminine Face of God*, and *The Three Faces of Sarah*. I try to meditate in the quiet space on the second floor. And still I think I am missing something.

I have no spiritual fiber in me."

"You're crazy, Mavis. What are you talking about? You are clearly a spiritual human being. The problem is that you don't know it yet."

Lydia dreams of spending time at a monastic retreat. Her spiritual journey has taken her from the rigor of a High Anglican Church through the progressive portals of a Unitarian congregation. She finally settled for a middle course, the United Church of Canada.

I too search for a spiritual home within my faith. I stray like the wandering Jew from synagogue to synagogue: First Nareyever Egalitarian Synagogue, Beth Tzedec Congregation, Darchei Noam Reconstructionist Synagogue, Oraynu Community for Secular Humanistic Judaism, Kolel Centre for Liberal Jewish Learning. I am seeking perfect harmony of form and content — traditional form and ritual, contemporary theology and text. I want to be wrapped in the melodies of my childhood and wear the prayer shawl of mystery and holiness. I want the beautiful sound of Hebrew. I want to be swept away by the rhythm of swaying bodies, to and fro in an ecstatic trance of religious outpouring. I want to chant the words of my ancestors and feel a union with that community.

But I am a woman. I too want to be given the opportunity for an *aliyah*. I want to be included in a *minyan*. I want to honor the names of the matriarchs as well as the patriarchs. I want to create new rituals to mark Rosh Chodesh, the new moon of each month. I too want to feel the goddess within me.

One of my friends says that I am searching for the impossible. Another says that I must not give up on my search. Lacan says you must not give up on your desires. What is my desire?

Debra, a childhood friend from Montreal who now lives in Toronto, shares in my struggles. She has sung in a synagogue choir for over ten years. "I cheat," she says softly. "I go to synagogue to sing, but I silently question my devotion."

Debra and I share similar religious backgrounds. She has explored Judaism, Taoism, and Buddhism. Now she is a student of S. N. Goenka, studying vipassana meditation. Debra explains that vipassana has nothing to do with any organized religion or with sectarianism. *Vipassana* means "seeing things as they really are," self-purification by self-observation. It promises no cures for physical or mental disease. Vipassana is an attempt to deal with the universal problems of greed, hatred, and ignorance.

Twice a year, Debra drives to Shelburne Falls, Massachusetts, for a ten-day retreat. The retreat's code of discipline is strict: abstinence from killing, stealing, sexual activity, telling lies, and all intoxicants. Noble Silence is observed for the entire period. I love the idea of silence of the body, mind, and speech. I imagine Debra, elegant and holy in the requisite simple, modest attire. I see her meditating in her room or in the Great Hall. I follow her as she moves through the center, being in silence. I try to imagine my capacity for such discipline.

• • •

The Bruce Trail winds 782 kilometers through Ontario, from Niagara north to Tobermory, at the tip of the Bruce Peninsula. It is the oldest and longest marked hiking trail in the world.

Lawlor and I begin a slow ascent to the lookout on Skinner's Bluff. We leave behind the white birch forest and the muddy waters of the Slough of Despond. As we quietly work our way through the undergrowth, following the blazes to the view of Colpoy's Bay, we carefully step over roots gnarled into sculptures. We push forward until we reach the height of land. On our right, steep cliffs form a sheer drop to Georgian Bay; on our left, the trail winds inland in serpentine patterns.

We stop, mesmerized by the view. Glacier-deposited boulders protrude. Turkey vultures circle above the trail. The sun reflects the colors of Canadian autumn behind us — russet, brown, orange, ocher — the shades of Mother Earth at the height of her glory.

"Biodiversity at its finest," Lawlor laughs, removing his pack to make a seat. "Life forms — nature's bounty. It doesn't get any better than this."

I undo my jacket and settle on an old-growth cedar root. I form my fingers into the shape of a camera. "*Click*. I've got you. Captured the moment, recorded the memory. I want to hold on to this forever."

Lawlor's expression changes. "That's the problem," he says, becoming serious. "Nothing is forever. We get too attached to things. The Diamond Sutra says that all things that appear in this world are transient, so if you view all appearances as non-appearances, then you will understand the true nature of everything. That means that everything is changing constantly. The cause of suffering is trying to hold on to something."

He stops, turns away, and then continues, "That's it. As soon as we get attached to something, we suffer because we can't hold on to it. It's like life. Attachment to life causes pain at the thought of death, because we are trying to hold on to something we can't have."

"Okay, so how does that help me with my work with cancer patients? How do you tell people who are dying of a vicious, relentless, nasty disease that they are too attached to life?"

I feel myself getting heated, my eyes beginning to tingle, when Lawlor responds, "Well, in a way, all explanations are just explanations, just words. From my own experience, nothing prepares you for the inevitability of pain from illness and the suffering that follows. No one truly understands why we are born or why we die or the way we die. When we are healthy, we ignore those questions. A meditation practice forces us to examine these mysteries and allows the clenched fist of our fear of death to open a little."

"Freud said that there is no resolution around the issue of death, that one can never come to terms with one's own mortality."

"I guess that's a major difference of opinion. Look, Mave, I'm not saying this is easy stuff. This is a lifetime effort. Another way of looking at it is to ask the question, 'Who is suffering, who is the *I* that is suffering?' The self is just an image, an illusion, maya.

"Take a candle, for example. You watch the flame, and even though it stays constant, the candle keeps changing its form, becoming smaller and smaller as it burns. When it comes to ourselves, we can't imagine another form. Our ego refuses to acknowledge this. The self, the ego, wants to hang on to the identity it has created for itself, so it struggles to maintain it, unchanging and constant. No matter how powerful the intellectual explanations, the words, or the questions, the ego is able to deflect the logic of the intellect. The only way to break through this is to transcend or get beyond the words. Through meditation, you come to understand who is suffering. You see how fragile the self-image really is. But, Mave, meditation is only one path to take."

I struggle to understand. I wade through the words. But Zen is "before words." Zen is "don't-know mind." I visualize one of my groups in front of me, each person cocooned in his or her own skin, an envelope of flesh. How do I say "We all die, only you are going to die sooner. But don't worry, you're not dying, you're just changing form"?

According to Judeo-Christian sources, there are alternative views. In the Book of Job, there is insistence on a response from God. Job's question demands an answer. Why the injustice? Why the suffering? He demands explanation. Yet is death part of that injustice? Or is death truly a part of life that requires no explanation, that simply is?

I realize that I do not believe in a personal god. I do not turn to God in personal prayers. I do not ask God for mercy or relief from suffering. I do not follow the 613 laws of my religion.

I do believe in a universal life force. Instead of "God," I whisper the words "great mystery" and I am calmed. I visualize a universal life force connecting me with all other sentient beings. And I believe in the importance of ritual — the need to celebrate festivals, to commemorate important life events, to inaugurate celebrations in order to create memories for the future. And I believe in the tribal urge to live in a community. My community begins with my family, but extends into my community of friends, colleagues, and acquaintances.

I am lost in my thoughts until Lawlor's voice pulls me out of myself. "Hey there, what happened? We were having a magical moment a little while ago. Let's move on."

• • •

> *Resilience* (ri-ZI-liens), 1626. 1. The (or an) act of rebounding or springing back; rebound, recoil. 2. Elasticity; the power of resuming to the original shape or position after bending, compression, etc. *Resiliency* (ri-ZI-lien-si), 1668. 1. Tendency to rebound or recoil. 2. = *resilience* 2, 1835. 3. Buoyancy, power of recoil, 1857.
>
> SHORTER OXFORD ENGLISH DICTIONARY

The graduate metastatic group is dwindling. Active illness, sickness, death. Selma calls me at my office and says she can no longer handle the group. "I can't take any more bad news right now."

Louise is in palliative care. Nathalie's surgery was not successful; her liver cancer has returned, metastasized to her spine. Terry calls me to say that Esther is back at home, then she does not complete her thoughts; there are no more treatment options open for her. Suzanne tells me at the end of a meeting that she needs time out from "cancer and the group." Tove has been rushed to emergency; she has not been able to keep food down for over a week.

Cancer is merciless. It does not let up. Sometimes I wonder if soon anyone will be left in the graduate group.

I break all the rules of therapy. I call Tove, Nathalie, Barbara,

Esther. I send flowers to Lynn, Sheila, Marcia, and James. I pray nightly, against my principles, for the peace of mind to continue my work. I pray nightly for peace of mind and body for everyone.

A few weeks later, Lynn dies, Esther dies, Tove dies. Bad things come in threes.

Who believes in miraculous recovery? Where are the miracles in my group? Nathalie died as she lived, fighting, resisting. Preeya died peacefully, praying, accepting.

Michael Lerner is founder and president of Commonweal in Bolinas, California, and a co-founder of the Commonweal Cancer Help program. I first saw him in a documentary on PBS in the *Healing and the Mind* series. In the book from the series, in a chapter entitled "Wounded Healers," he writes,

> There aren't a lot of cures. Documented spontaneous remissions from cancer are reported in the medical literature, and these cases are a very important field of research. There are hundreds of articles describing probably thousands of cases in the medical literature, but if you look at the individual level, and study the likelihood that someone with a metastatic breast cancer or lung cancer or pancreatic cancer will, by his or her own inner resources be able to reverse this cancer and have it go away forever — well, that's a very steep slope. So the more interesting question is not "Is this cancer going to disappear completely?" but "Is more than an improved quality of life going to take place as a result of healing interventions?" The answer to that is, we really don't know.

I read that resilience is the ability to recover from loss without succumbing to suffering, as if nothing but an elastic rebound were involved, as if suffering were not an inevitable byproduct of life.

• • •

I remember the first time I thought the moon was following me. I was walking along the sidewalk and turned to face my dad, who was saying, "Look at the moon. The man in the moon is smiling."

I looked up to see a shimmering white plate suspended in the night's darkness. Then I looked away and continued counting my steps.

"I think he is smiling at you," my dad said, and I turned around to catch the moon's shift of position.

"The moon is following me, the moon is following me," I repeated out loud.

A week later, I shared my secret with Claudia Larsden, a playmate who lived down the street. In typical five-year-old fashion, we experimented at the first opportunity. Our brief excursion into physics nearly ended our friendship as we fought over exactly which of us the moon was following.

Many years later, I learned about perspective, illusions, and the power of thoughts. I also learned about the sun, the moon, the stars, the earth, and the universe. None of this convinced me enough about the power of illusion to satisfy my curiosity, or made me stop to question the meanings we create as we lead our lives.

As I got older, I discovered other mysteries, other experiences that massage our souls and transform us into mystics and poets and artists. It was then that I discovered the limitations of knowledge and explanations. Can the world ever offer an explanation of itself? Do explanations help in the presence of human suffering?

The scientific tradition of the Western world is based on a rational paradigm associated with the philosophical tradition of logical positivism. It is a science of observation, measurement, and proof. Our Western view of medicine is based on an interventionist model that grew out of this same paradigm. As a result, the medical model of treatment is prescriptive — do this, take that. Doctors are men in white coats who make things better, who "fix it." Even in grief-work there is a tendency to describe the stages and phases of grief, with a diagnosis of pathology for the person who does not fit the paradigm.

Professionals are uncomfortable about accepting that things cannot always be neatly described, that there are not always solutions and answers to the problems presented. Particularly in the mental health field, patients make demands on professionals to make them "feel better," and too easily the professional slips into the role of authority or expert who tries to provide the fix-it service being requested.

I have reconsidered this focus. My desire is to help others explore the meaning of cancer in their lives, to help them figure out how best to get through the day. At the same time, I need to explore my own issues so that I can continue to find new ways of being with others on this journey.

Joan Halifax, a Zen master in Santa Fe, once said in an interview,

> Rather than a guide, a therapist, I feel like a traveler, a pilgrim myself. Whether we know it or not, we're all traveling on the same trackless way through the forest to a place we've never visited before. Teachers can tell you things; professionals can listen; maps can give you a feeling about the shape of the territory. But it is only through personal experience that you truly learn.

EPILOGUE

The room is cool today; there has been a dramatic shift in the weather. Fall is so unpredictable. I orient myself to the unlit room. Today I am beginning a new twelve-week group for men and women with metastatic cancer.

When all ten people on the list have assembled, I begin. "My name is Mavis and I will be facilitating this twelve-week group. Before introducing ourselves, we will start with a brief relaxation visualization exercise."

I hear the breathing in the room deepen and I feel my pulse slow down. I speak slowly, "Okay, then. Just begin to turn your attention inwards and focus on your breathing . . ."

When I draw the group back to the room after the exercise, we begin the introductions.

"My name is Rose. I am fifty-two years old. I have soft-tissue carcinoma in the pelvic area and it has recurred in the pelvic area and metastasized to the lungs and pancreas . . ."

"My name is Nadia. I am a family physician. I found a lump on my breast. When it was diagnosed, it had already metastasized to the liver and spine . . ."

"My name is Arlene. I was diagnosed with breast cancer ten years ago. It has now spread to the liver . . ."

"My name is Jacquie. I am fifty-eight years old. I was diagnosed with lung cancer, which has metastasized to the bone and brain. I am a non-smoker with no family history of cancer . . ."

"My name is Walter. I was diagnosed with lung cancer, which has metastasized to the bones. I was a smoker. Four years ago, I was diagnosed and treated for prostate cancer. I think that was the dress rehearsal . . ."

"My name is Elly. I was diagnosed with Stage III ovarian cancer. My doctor told me I am buying time . . ."

"My name is Paula. I was diagnosed with breast cancer in '91. It recurred in the same breast in '98. In the fall of 2000, it metastasized to the spine and frontal lobe . . ."

"My name is Robin. I am thirty-eight years old. Two years ago, I was diagnosed with breast cancer. In October it metastasized to the lungs. I have five children, aged four to thirteen . . ."

"My name is Grace. I was diagnosed with breast cancer in '99 with no lymph node involvement. A year later, it had spread to my sternum and bones. I am divorced with two children aged ten and four . . ."

"My name is Helen. I have breast cancer, which has metastasized to the lungs, liver, and bones. One month ago, my doctor told me there is no further treatment he can recommend for me . . ."

I am never ready for this group.

* * *

Transitions. The transition between work and play, between day and night, between weekday and weekend. Transitioning: a sewing machine that stitches together the pattern of the day, an invisible seam binding the moments of our lives.

I leave the office. I leave behind the wingback chair, the silhouette of tulips on the wall, the overcrowded shelves of books. I leave the muted tones and pastel shades. I close the door and walk out into the autumn chill.

Lawlor is out of town. I have a weekend to myself. I resist the temptation to call Lydia, Ninna, Debra, or the other women with whom I share my free moments. Instead I decide to prepare a quiet meal and relax in front of the television.

I step lightly, out of one world and into another.

Lawlor has returned from his conference. He tells me that he was talking to some friends about my work at Wellspring and found himself confronted with that same difficult question: "How does Mavis deal with all that pain, suffering, and loss?" He tells me that he floundered about, trying to respond to this significant question in my "voice."

As he recounts the incident, I realize that the question no longer provokes a sensation of despair in my stomach. I do not feel my muscles tighten or my heart speed up. I can now see what my experiences have taught me.

I have learned that suffering — be it physical, mental, or both — is an inevitable part of life. And I know that illness causes suffering, not only for the person with the diagnosis but for a whole community of friends and relatives.

I have learned that we must all face our end, and for some people this end may be sooner than for others. I have learned that for some, the inevitability of death will be a terror that weighs heavily on them and causes a storm of bitterness and outrage that lasts to the final breath of life. But I also know that, for others, fear of death can resolve itself into peaceful acceptance and appreciation of a life lived.

I have learned that the human spirit is remarkably resilient, creative, and spirited in the face of illness and death, and that life takes on a heightened dimension of awareness in these circumstances.

I have learned that I will always be saddened by the pain and suffering that some patients endure, and by the loss of so many special people with whom I have come in contact.

And finally, I have learned that each day is a blessing and that one day it will be my turn. And I hope that when that day comes, there will be others who will listen to my story, my fears, and my wishes — not to force a resolution, but with acceptance and peace.

BIBLIOGRAPHY

American Cancer Society. <www.cancer.org.au/act/index.htm>

Canadian Cancer Society. *Canadian Cancer Statistics* (Toronto: National Cancer Institute of Canada, 1999).

Dollinger, Martin, and Ernest Rosenbaum, eds. *Everyone's Guide to Cancer Therapy* (Toronto: Somerville House Publishing, 1992).

Frähm, Anne, and David Frähm. *A Cancer Battle Plan* (Colorado Springs: Piñon Press, 1992).

Freud, Sigmund. "Feminine Sexuality" (1931). In *Standard Edition of the Complete Psychological Works of Sigmund Freud,* translated and edited by J. Strachey (London: Hogarth Press, 1953-1974).

Goldstein, Elyse. *ReVisions* (Toronto: Key Porter Books, 1998).

Halifax, Roshi Joan. "A Cool, Clear Wind" <www.upaya.org/roshi/Interview.html>

Herman, Nini. *Too Long a Child: The Mother-Daughter Dyad* (London: Free Association Books, 1989).

Kiple, Kenneth, ed. *The Cambridge History of Human Disease* (Cambridge: Cambridge University Press, 1983).

Lerner, Michael. "Healing." In *Healing and the Mind,* edited by Bill Moyers (New York: Doubleday, 1993).

Love, Susan. *Dr. Susan Love's Breast Book* (New York: Addison-Wesley, 1995).

Morrow, Susan Brind. *The Names of Things* (New York: Riverhead Books, 1997).

Myss, Caroline. *Why People Don't Heal and How They Can* (New York: Three Rivers Press / Crown Publishers, 1997).

Nasio, Juan-David. *Five Lessons on the Psychoanalytic Theory of Jacques Lacan,* translated by David Pettigrew and Francois Raffoul (New York: State University of New York Press, 1998).

Ontario Breast Cancer Information Exchange Partnership. *A Guide to Unconventional Cancer Therapies* (Toronto: Ontario Breast Cancer Information Exchange Partnership, 1994).

Ponder, Catherine. *The Healing Secrets of the Ages* (Los Angeles, CA: DeVorss, 1969).

Remen, Rachel Naomi. "Wholeness." In *Healing and the Mind,* edited by Bill Moyers (New York: Doubleday, 1993).

Rothenberg, Beno. *Sinai* (Berne: Kummerly and Frey, 1979).

Schmitt, Waldo. *Crustaceans* (Ann Arbor, MI: University of Michigan Press, 1965).

Trepp, Leo. *The Complete Book of Jewish Observance* (New York: Behrman House / Simon & Schuster, 1980).

Weiseltier, Leon. *Kaddish* (New York: Alfred A. Knopf, 1998).

Yalom, Irvin. *The Theory and Practice of Group Psychotherapy* (New York: Basic Books, 1985).